AN INTRODUCTION TO LIFESTYLE MANAGEMENT

Participant's Workbook

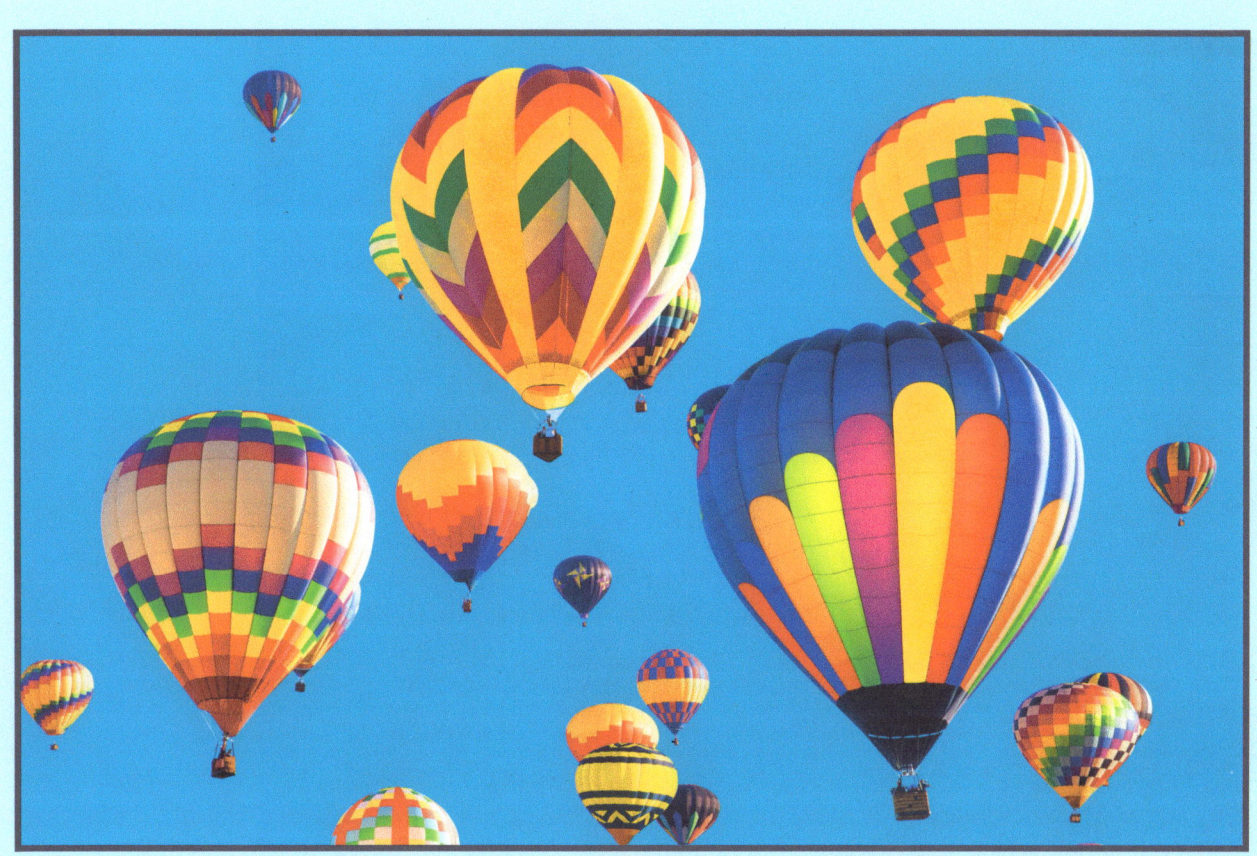

Dr Anja Morris-Paxton

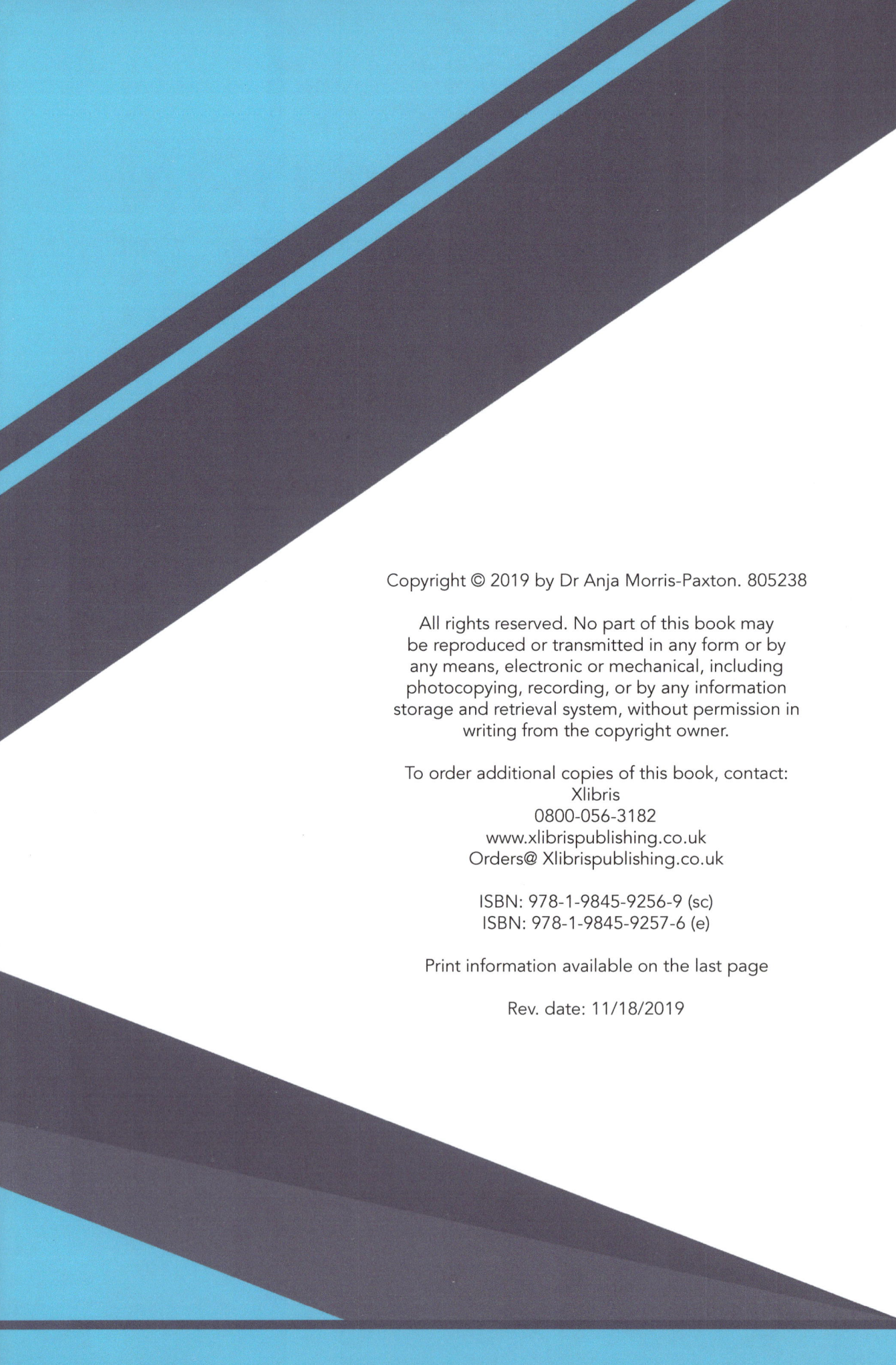

To order additional copies of this book, contact:
Xlibris
0800-056-3182
www.xlibrispublishing.co.uk
Orders@ Xlibrispublishing.co.uk

ISBN: 978-1-9845-9256-9 (sc)
ISBN: 978-1-9845-9257-6 (e)

Print information available on the last page

Rev. date: 11/18/2019

AN INTRODUCTION TO LIFESTYLE MANAGEMENT

Participant's Workbook

Anja Morris-Paxton

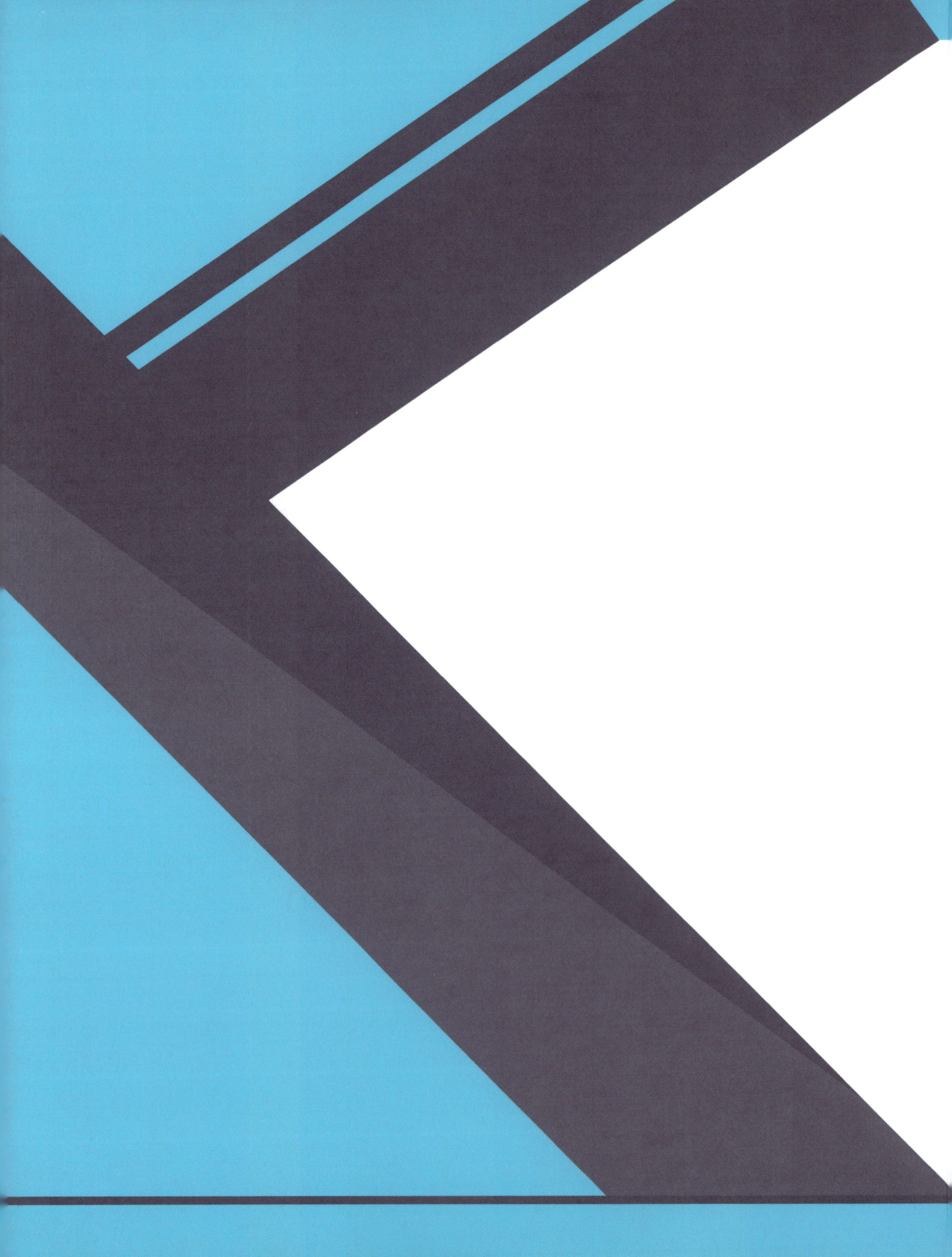

A Facilitated Course Designed for Further and Higher Education Foundational Learning

Adult and Community Learning

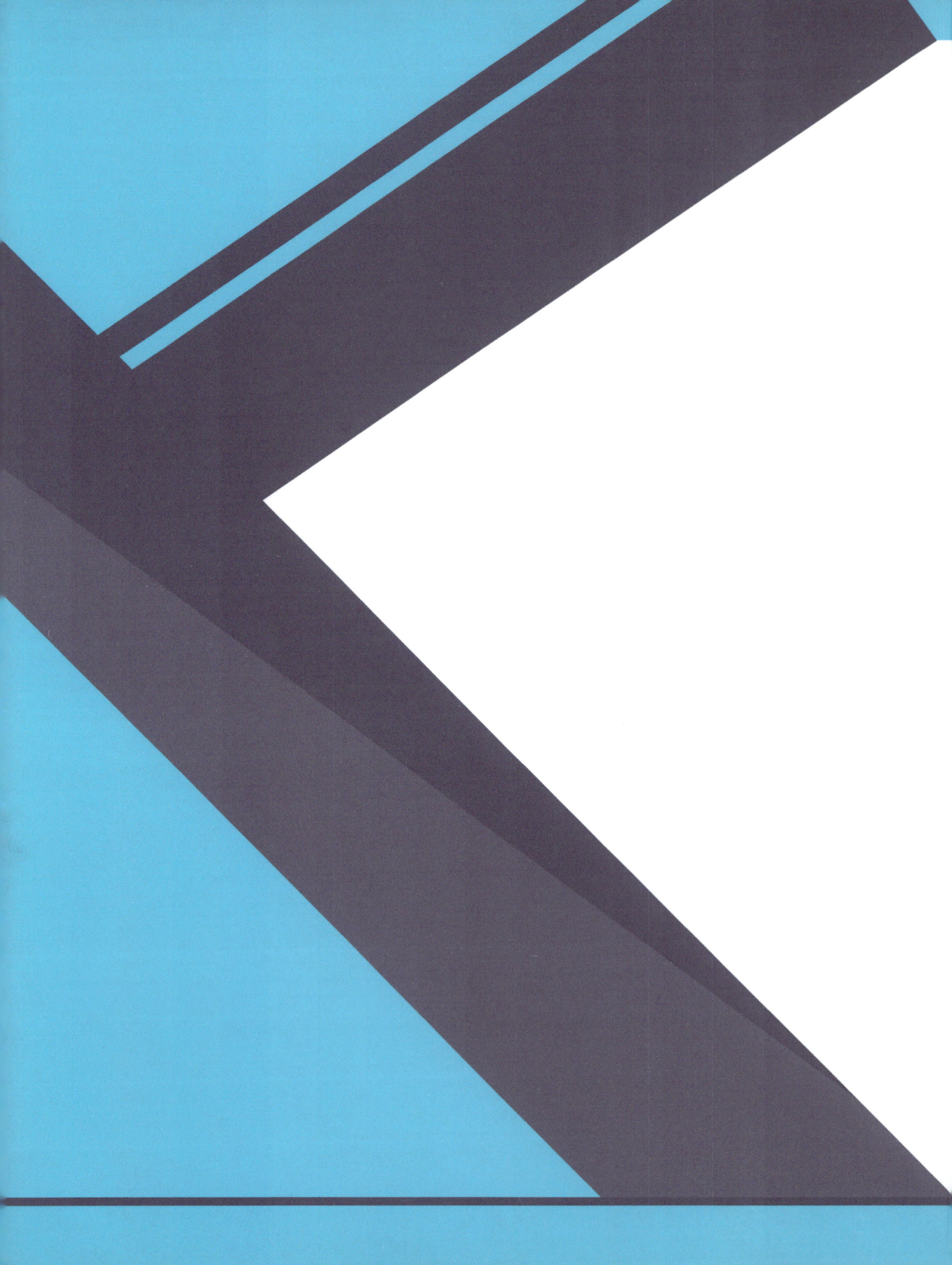

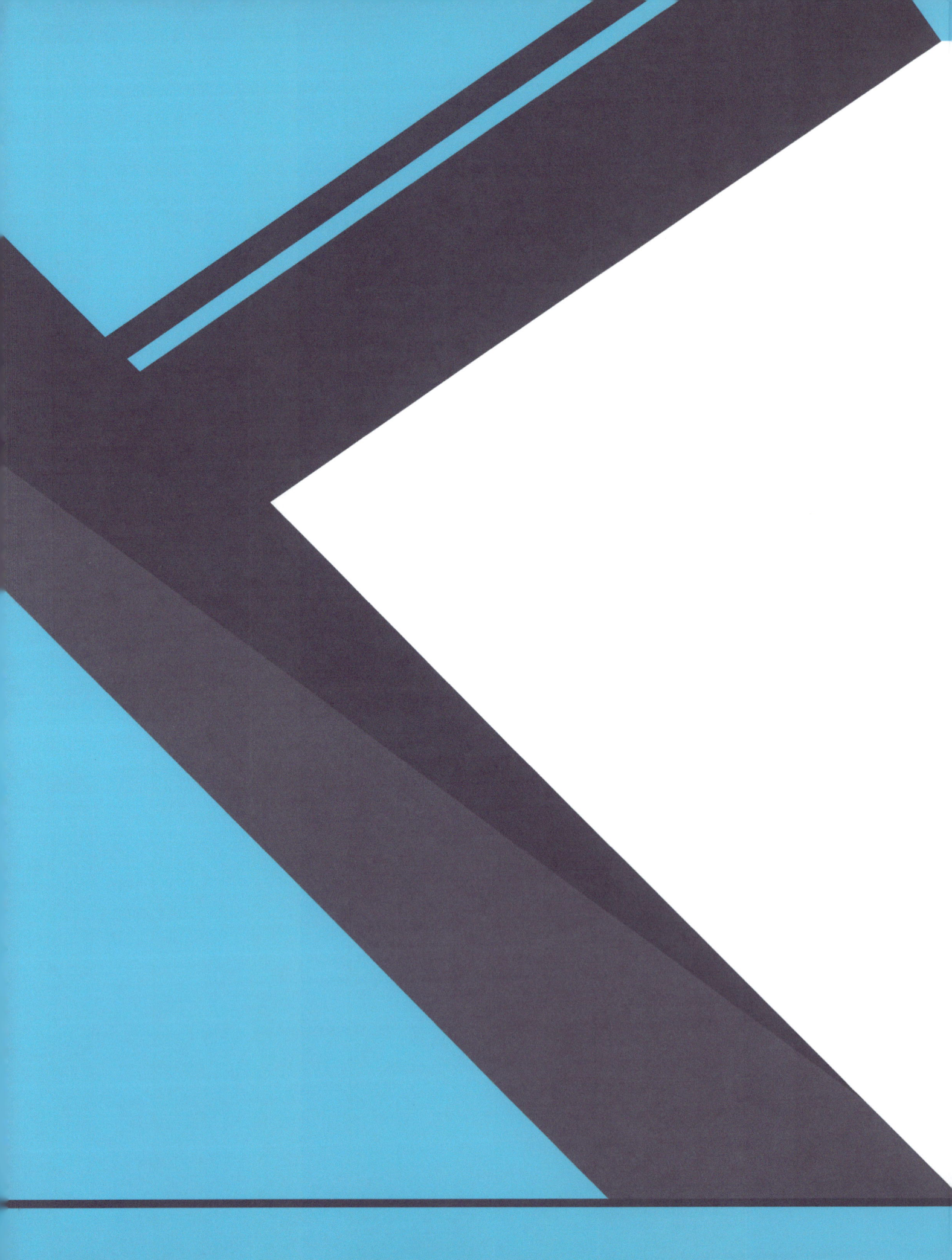

Basic Information About This Programme

Programme Title   : An Introduction to Lifestyle Management

Programme Level   : Further and Foundational Higher Education

Adult and Community Learning

(ACL)

Hours Required   : 36 hours facilitated learning

Programme Length   : 12 learning sessions

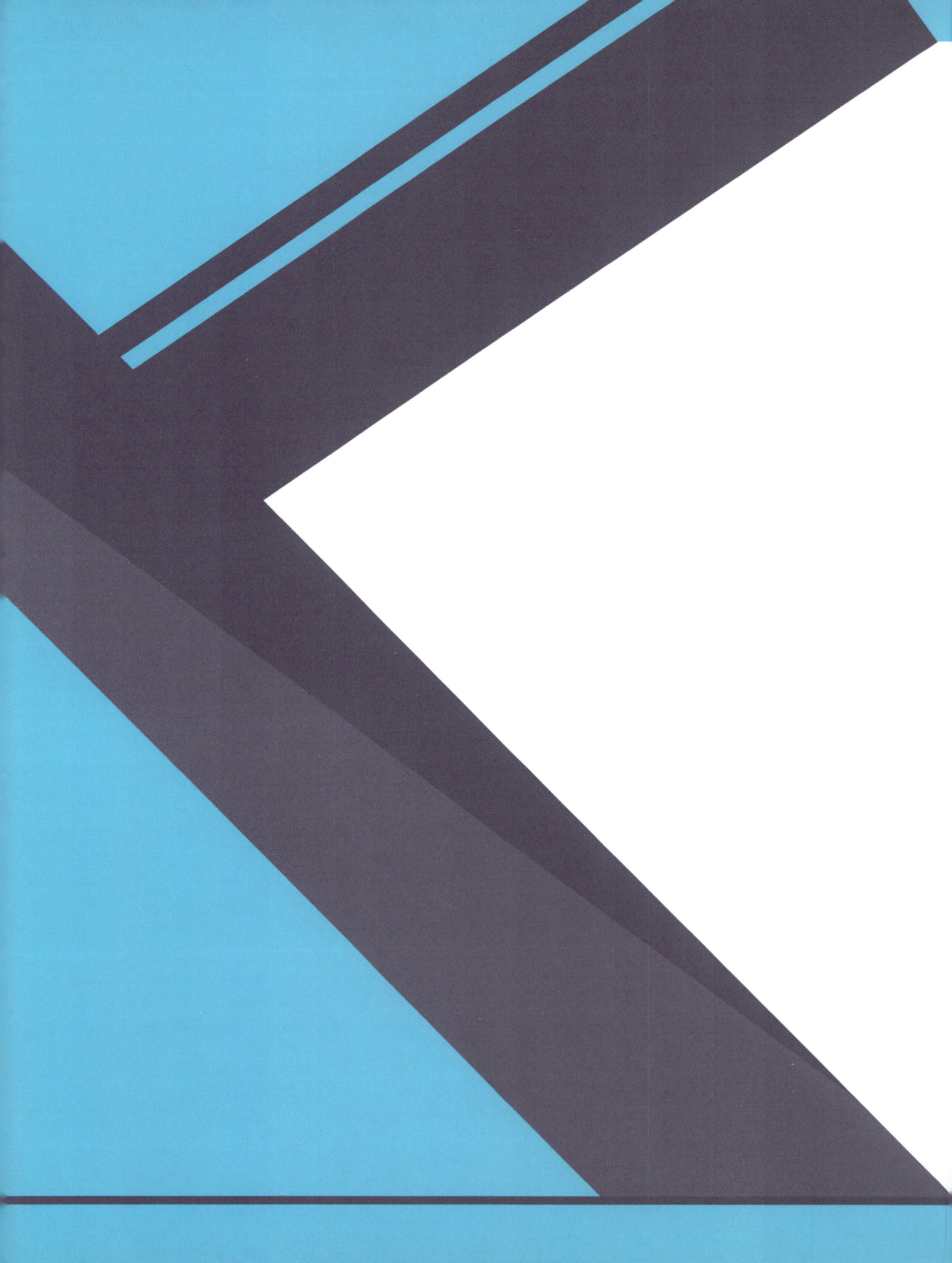

CONTENTS

PROGRAMME REVIEWERS

Malcolm J Dedman

Malcolm Dedman graduated from Brunel University with an Honours Degree in Technology (Applied Physics) and worked for more than 20 years in the sound technology and engineering industry, where he was responsible for several research and development projects. Malcolm has always had a keen interest in both music and health and later graduated with distinction from Thames Valley University with a Masters in Music Composition. Malcolm brings with him skills in reviewing, proofing and editing research reports and technical manuals and has reviewed the material in this course for literary content, accuracy, and presentation. In addition, he has taken the stance of a programme participant in his critique of the appropriateness and usefulness of the content.

Hanna van Lingen

Hanna van Lingen is a Counselling Psychologist and works as a Senior Student Counsellor at the Nelson Mandela University in Port Elizabeth, South Africa. Her doctoral research topic related to higher education student wellness. Her role in student counselling includes the development and facilitation of workshops and training sessions for students and colleagues, as well as the coordination of the student counselling centre's psychosocial development and wellness programmes and services. Hanna was one of the founder members of the former Wellness Council of Southern Africa (WELLCOSA, 2000-2008), and one of the developers of the Wellness Questionnaire for Higher Education (WQHE). She maintains an academic involvement – she has lectured on a part-time basis for more than 20 years (amongst others, in Lifestyle Management), and has been involved with several wellness-related postgraduate research projects as supervisor or co-supervisor. Hanna reviewed this course from her perspective as both a practitioner and an academic, looking at course content, its research base, and the presentation format of the training sessions.

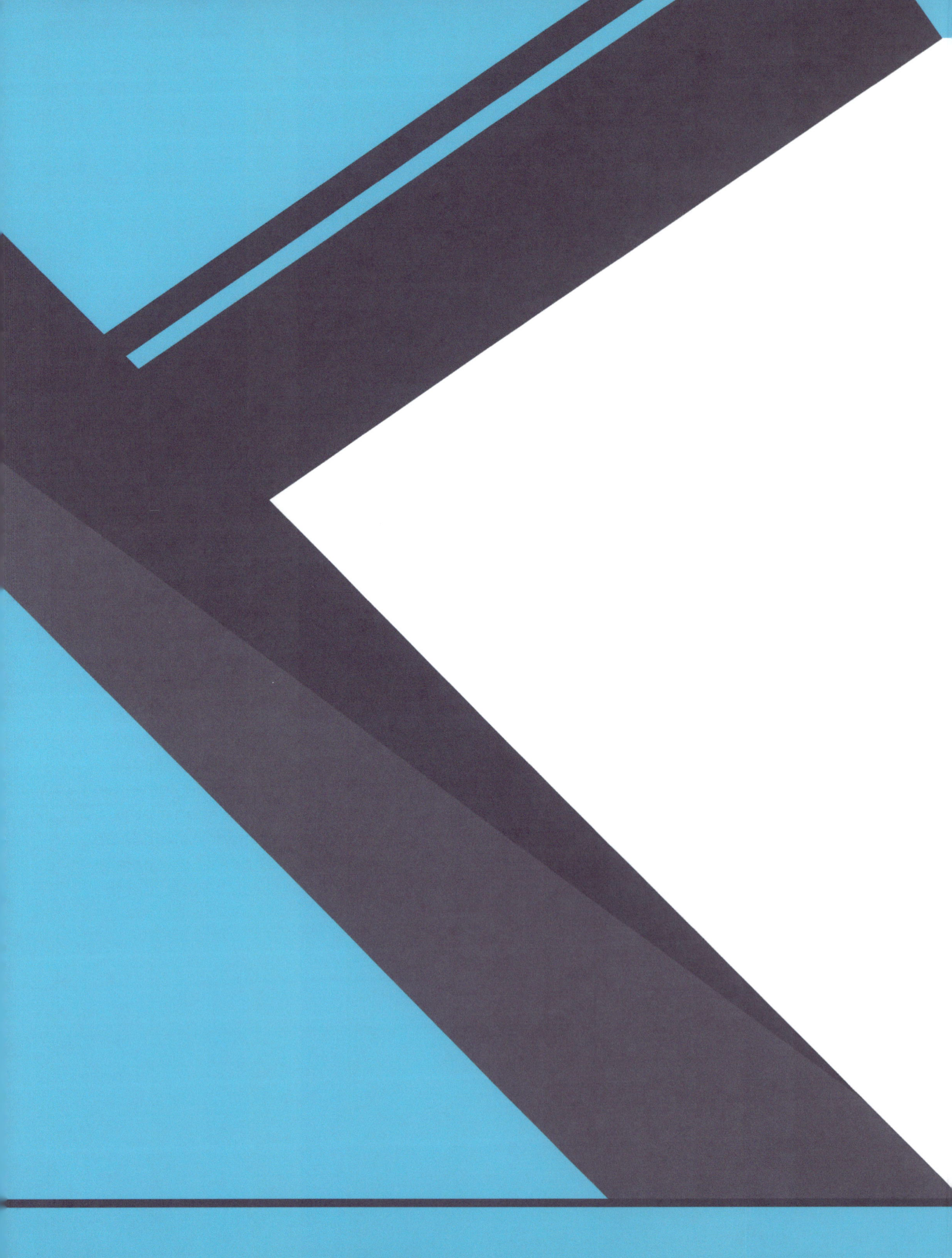

REVIEW OF AN INTRODUCTION TO LIFESTYLE MANAGEMENT

The Introduction to Lifestyle Management Programme is the second programme to be designed and authored by Anja Morris-Paxton, and it focuses on helping the participants to make improvements to and to manage their lifestyle. Following on from the Introduction to Concepts of Nutrition, this programme includes a summary of nutrition, as well as including many other topics that are designed to help the individual to maintain a healthy and well-balanced lifestyle.

Like the first programme, much information is widely available for many of the topics covered, but those in search of the relevant facts will often be faced with conflicting and sometimes controversial information. Dr Morris-Paxton, however, takes the same scientific approach as before, frequently referencing latest and verifiable research that supports the information she presents.

In addition to a brief summary of nutrition, so essential for managing our health, topics included in the twelve learning sessions are: discussions about the use of cigarettes, alcohol and medication; the benefits of exercise and movement; the importance of water, air and sunlight; a study of the effect of bacteria and parasites; how to know ourselves and how we relate to others; how to manage stress; a discussion on the importance of our mind and how we think; and finally, an examination of our beliefs. It can, therefore, be seen that these topics cover the wide spectrum of physical, mental, emotional and spiritual disciplines, a holistic approach that is so essential to an improved and fulfilling quality of life.

In writing the programme, Dr Morris-Paxton recognises that there is not one solution for everyone, but by means of exercises, quizzes and discussion sessions, participants are encouraged to decide for themselves how best to apply the information provided, so that they may draw on their cultural influences and personal tastes.

The knowledge gained from this programme is essential to everyone, as it aims to bring together the latest research findings so that the individual can make better and informed choices as to how they can make lifestyle improvements tailored to their own individual needs. The programme is not only a 'must' for everyone, whatever their background, but also the participation is a most enjoyable and informative experience.

Malcolm Dedman, B Tech (Hons), MMus

I had the opportunity to view the *Introduction to Lifestyle Management: Facilitator's Handbook* by Dr Morris-Paxton. In terms of programme content, I found the holistically focused, twelve-session Lifestyle Management programme to be comprehensive in its scope. Topics related to physical lifestyle management are extensively covered, such as nutrition, movement, and substance use. Psychosocial aspects of lifestyle management are also included in the coursework, with topics such as stress management, social relationships, emotions, thoughts, and spirituality being addressed. Each session is appropriately titled in a user-friendly way; for example, "Mastering the Mayhem" for the session on managing stress. Each chapter presents clearly formulated learning outcomes and includes carefully researched and referenced texts.

In addition to a lecturing format being used, there is a strong emphasis on experiential learning – quizzes, exercises and group discussions are included, making the material suitable for participants with different learning styles. Each of the twelve sessions is concluded with a group discussion, where participants have the opportunity to apply their new knowledge and insights gained through the session, resulting in the consolidation of their learning. The active participation allows learners to be not only passive recipients, but co-constructors of their own learning experience and its outcomes. True to the spirit of experiential learning, the course content is not prescriptive, but allows participants to determine for themselves what learning they want to "take home" from each exercise or session.

Dr Morris-Paxton follows a consultative approach in the development of her learning and teaching materials, seeking feedback from her peers, trainers/facilitators and course participants alike, as well as staying abreast of new research publications. The result is a constantly evolving and relevant curriculum – one that is responsive to new subject knowledge as well as to the needs of the learners and the community.

Hanna van Lingen
MA (Counselling Psychology), DPhil (Psychology)

INTRODUCTION

Welcome

Welcome to the Introduction to Lifestyle Management Programme. The aim of this programme is to facilitate a unique learning environment in which you, as the participant, can develop the underpinning knowledge and skills required for the prevention of ill-health through appropriate lifestyle management. The material has been developed where possible from academically accepted reference books and peer-reviewed research papers, as well as the expertise and experience of the author.

The principles of lifestyle management and the methods applied to provide new knowledge and understanding in this programme are holistic. This means that the physical, psychological, social, emotional and affective context in which people conduct their lives within their own surroundings has been considered. As this programme is facilitated, you will be guided through your learning. The nature of facilitated learning programmes is that participants are encouraged to make their own decisions and to help one another as a group. The nature of participation is to gain the knowledge, understanding and skills that you feel can benefit you most.

All the learning sessions are of equal length and are conducted with most of the new knowledge being given in the first half of the session. The role of the facilitator is to lead the sessions and help each group with the quick quizzes that are interspersed between each section of learning and the learning together activities. In addition, your facilitator will chair the discussions in the second part of each session. Creating this programme has been interesting and enjoyable. It is my hope that the result is an equally interesting and enjoyable venture into an easier and more manageable world for you .

Anja Morris-Paxton

OVERVIEW OF THE PROGRAMME

Practical lifestyle management encompasses two kinds of knowledge and ability. The first is a knowledge and understanding of the components of health that we require as human beings to work, learn, socialise and develop to be at our best. We need to develop an understanding of what they are and why they are beneficial. The second is the ability to use these components together, to acquire lifestyle management skills in the context of our individual lives, to obtain the maximum benefits.

This programme looks at lifestyle management from a holistic point of view in that it not only gives the facts about the components of a lifestyle that bring about or prevent disease but also explores ways to use the physical, social, mental and affective / spiritual components of living to our own benefit. The programme encompasses twelve facilitated learning sessions which look at the spectrum of physical, mental, emotional and spiritual disciplines that can detract from or enhance, the process of building long term health and well-being.

Aims of the Programme

1. To develop the ability to recognise the essential components of health and, to appreciate how the management of these components detract from, or enhance, long term health and well-being.
2. To explore the choices available to the individual in each component of lifestyle within the context of one's family and community life.
3. To develop the ability to prevent problems arising from incorrect management of lifestyle habits and, the confidence to create and apply corrective solutions in the context of one's own environment.
4. To appraise the tools that can be used to plan a diet, engage in movement, utilise medication and professional assistance, interact appropriately with others and develop a healthy self-image.

Learning Outcomes

When participants have completed this programme, they should be able to:

1. Demonstrate knowledge of the essential components of health care and the consequences of mismanagement of these components.

2. Appraise both the short- and long-term benefits of good management of the components of lifestyle.
3. Demonstrate an understanding of a variety of practical, beneficial mechanisms that may be applicable within the various components of an individual lifestyle programme.
4. Make appropriate individual choices within each component of lifestyle within the context of one's own environment.
5. Use a variety of tools to plan a diet, engage in movement, utilise medication and professional assistance, interact appropriately with others and develop a healthy self-image to meet one's individual requirements within the context of one's own environment.
6. Demonstrate the ability and the confidence to apply corrective solutions to problems of lifestyle using a variety of tools and management approaches

THE LEARNING SESSIONS

<u>Learning Session One: The constituents of a healthy lifestyle and the place of lifestyle management in the prevention of disease</u>

This session covers the importance of lifestyle management and, introduces you to the individual constituents of a healthy lifestyle; nutrition; avoiding substance abuse and the appropriate use of medication; exercise; the importance of hydration and the use of sunlight and fresh air; controlling bacteria and parasites as well as social relationships, self-esteem and the management of stress. We look at the role of these measures in the prevention of long-term ill health and how ignorance and abuse contribute to disease.

<u>Learning Session Two: Nutrition and lifestyle – the constituents of a good diet</u>

This session looks at the essential nutrients that we require for good health. These fall into two groups: The macronutrients, being carbohydrates fats and proteins, and the micronutrients, being vitamins and minerals. We look at the best forms of macronutrients, which ones are good for us and which are not and the food sources of both macronutrients and micronutrients. In addition, we discuss why we need certain nutrients and the adverse consequences of an inadequate and / or unbalanced diet.

<u>Learning Session Three: The colour wheel</u>

We discover in this session one of the tools we can use to create our own daily or weekly nutritional programme. 'The Colour Wheel' can be customised for one's own personal needs. We look at portion sizes, the timing of meals and snacks and an understanding of why breakfast is so important and how to get over the problem of early morning lack of appetite.

<u>Learning Session Four: Cigarettes and alcohol, the visible and hidden costs</u>

In this session, we discuss nicotine and what the physical, psychological and social effects of smoking are, from individual health risks to the economic and environmental risks. In addition, we look at the controversy surrounding 'responsible drinking', how much is enough, and how much is too much? We discuss whether alcohol is good for anything at all that we cannot obtain from other sources, and the real and hidden costs of drinking may be.

Learning Session Five: Pills and potions – the right way and the wrong way to use medication

In this session, we look at the correct way to use medication and seek professional health care advice, what one can do for oneself, and when it is appropriate to ask for assistance. We discuss the use and possible abuse of antibiotics, painkillers and over the counter remedies as well as complementary medicines and, how to understand and adhere to instructions. In addition, we review the growing problem of recreational substance abuse as well as addiction to both illegal, over the counter and prescribed medications.

Learning Session Six: Movement and health

We explore here the connection not only between exercise, movement and health but also between movement and self-expression. There are many ways in which one can engage with movement from traditional dancing to modern equipped gymnasiums, from team sport to home gardening. Some of the suggestions require membership of a club or gym and others are available free of charge and without obligation. We discuss the benefits of movement and discover ways in which each of us can find something we enjoy doing and motivate ourselves to continue.

Learning Session Seven: Environmental health

Here we look at the elements we need to survive, what they are, why they are essential and, most importantly, what they have to do with a programme on lifestyle management! Water, air and sunlight are essential to all growth, whether that of plants, animals or human beings. We discover why and how these are important to us. We look at the issue of adequate hydration, the quality of our air and the appropriate amount of sunlight necessary to health, and how to gain the maximum benefit with the minimum damage.

Learning Session Eight: The unwelcome guests

We share our environment internally and externally with both beneficial and harmful bacteria. We discuss what the most common bacteria and parasites are and where they come from. In addition, this session discusses how to eliminate or at least reduce the harmful elements while retaining the beneficial ones in the context of our relationship with the environment around us. Finally, we discuss the use of antibiotics and antibacterial cleansers when they are beneficial and when they may contribute to the problem.

Learning Session Nine: Intrapersonal and interpersonal – knowing yourself and getting to know others

Here we look inside at who we really are our potential for good and our value to the community and wider society. We view the issue of friendship and how we can be a friend to ourselves as opposed to our own worst enemy. We discuss the issue of going it alone, resisting peer pressure as well as the value of supporting and caring friendship with others. We ask ourselves what a true friend is and how can we become a true friend to someone else. Also, we view our interaction with others, the benefit of belonging to a group and being part of a successful democratic community.

Learning Session Ten: Mastering the mayhem

This session helps us to evaluate stress levels in one's life and to put the issues of concern into perspective. We look at values and priorities, how to organise ourselves, our time, and how to prioritise tasks in our daily lives. In addition, we discuss the emergencies, disasters and setbacks that occur in daily living. We view ways we can manage these, controlling the situation rather than being overwhelmed by it, and how to turn down responsibilities that are beyond our personal resources, without alienating those around us. Finally, we look at coping skills, how we can develop strengths through adversity, and how to create a contingency for possible future adversity.

Learning Session Eleven: Mind, mentality and the material

In this session, we look at the power of the mind, how our thoughts create emotions which, in turn, create chemical reactions in our body that affect our health and well-being. We look at the power of both negative and positive emotions and how to turn bad feelings into good energy. What do our priorities have to do with our health and well-being? We look at happiness and ask, is this fate or trait? There are differences in the health of happy and unhappy people, and we explore ways in which we can learn to be happy.

Learning Session Twelve: Faith and feeling, the place of belief and self-expression in health

In this final session, we view the presence (or absence), of the divine aspect of our lives and the power of faith. Does this play a role in our lives, and does it affect our health? We review some interesting scientific research on faith and health, the benefits of faith, and how to access spiritual strengths which you might not have realised you possessed. Self-expression can additionally be utilised to create health and well-being, and priorities can be re-defined. Finally, we look at utilising the power of using positive, creative thought, to benefit our health and well-being.

THE LEARNING SESSIONS

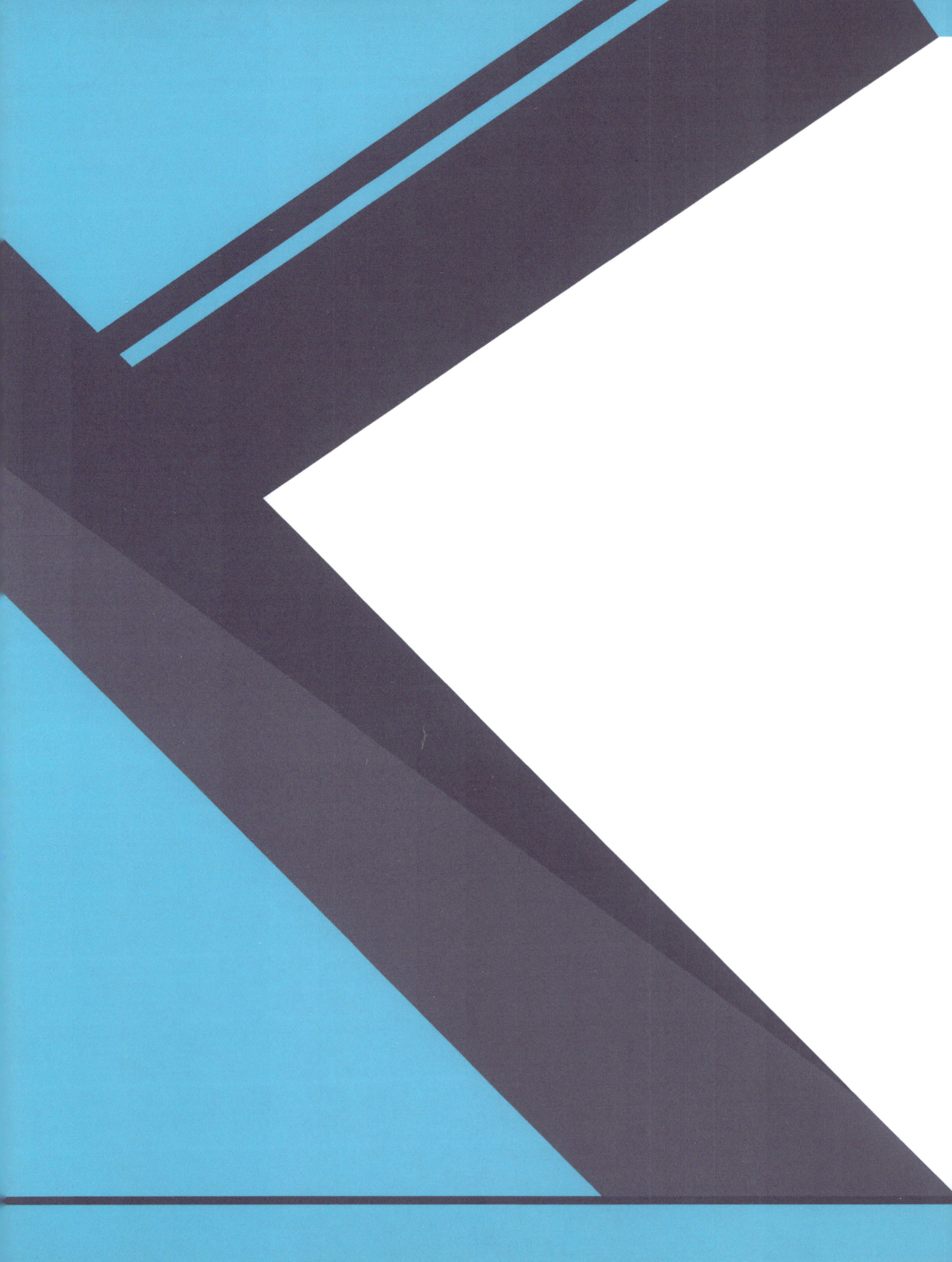

LEARNING SESSION ONE: THE CONSTITUENTS OF A HEALTHY LIFESTYLE AND THE PLACE OF LIFESTYLE MANAGEMENT IN THE PREVENTION OF DISEASE

Introduction

This session covers both the obvious and not so obvious differences between health and disease. In addition, the session covers the constituents of a healthy lifestyle and the importance of lifestyle management. Initially, we will look at the definitions of health and disease and how this has changed over the past few decades. We then look briefly at the causes of illness and its management and prevention. At this point, we come to our first learning together session where we engage in a little fun exercise with one another, in small groups.

We then move on to take a brief overview of the constituents of lifestyle, how these are divided into various categories that deal with physical, psychological, emotional and spiritual well-being. We see the breadth of what exactly this entails and take a brief look at some of the aspects of their management.

Quick quizzes are interspersed throughout the session before we finally look at just why managing one's lifestyle appropriately is important. The quality of life one has as an individual affects the community that surrounds us and the future quality of life for all. Our second learning together session is found at the end of this section. Finally, we come to our discussion session, and we look at the issue of peer pressure: how the opinions of others affect us and whether we are easily persuaded. Do we have difficulty in saying 'no' to others, or are we too stubborn to change our minds even when it might be for the better? We look at the influence of peer pressure on our confidence levels and the possibility of our future success.

Ice-Breaker Quiz

Let us look at the components of life and health and see how well we are doing and whether there is room for improvement:

A. Which of the following would you rate as having an impact on health?

Nutrition	Exercise	Sleep	Fresh Air	Stress Management
	Weight Control	Medication		Personal Hygiene
Regular Doctors' Visits		Dental Care	Faith	Sunshine
	Reducing Salt	Hobbies		Drinking Clean Water
Positive Outlook	Relaxation		Active Social Life	

B. Decide on the ten most important

C. Place your score of how well, on average, you are doing by each item on your list

Awesome! = 5   Good = 4   OK = 3   Poor = 2   Gross = 1

1. _____   6. _____

2. _____   7. _____

3. _____   8. _____

4. _____   9. _____

5._____   10. _____

Disease and Health: The Perceptions and the Reality

Disease has, for most of the history of mankind, been thought of predominantly as physical incapacitation due to injury, infection, or congenital deformity. Health has simply been the absence of such problems, freedom from pain and the ability to perform physical work. Merriam Webster defines health as the condition of an organism or one of its parts in which it performs its vital functions normally or properly: the state of being sound in body or mind; *especially*: freedom from physical disease and pain. Health maintenance is defined as the provision of comprehensive health care to individuals and families with limited referral to outside specialists [1]. Although limited in scope, for many years, this was the way in which health was principally thought of, in terms of **pathogenesis**, i.e. the process of how one becomes ill.

We have now moved on; the current focus is one of **salutogenesis**, the process by which one becomes well. Life has now progressed towards greater possibilities for achievement, and the concept of health has changed. The World Health Organisation (WHO) has defined health as ***The level of well-being that allows for the total fulfilment of the physical, psychological, educational and occupational potential of each individual*** [2].

Rather than referring to health or illness, we now embrace the salutogenesis of both individuals and populations when we refer to the ***'wellness arena'***. The wellness arena incorporates wellness consultants, the healthcare professions and disease prevention specialists; in addition to the manufacture of medicines, medicinal aids and meeting the clinical needs, lifestyle requirements and some of the relaxation and leisure provision (spa's hydro's and gymnasiums) of the population. Such services and professions are now referred to collectively as '***the wellness industry'***. The art of taking care of one's own health is about developing an understanding of life and a value for life that provides a basis for a sufficiently responsible way of living. This, in turn, promotes the development of self-confidence and the ability to solve problems [3].

One can no longer separate health and wealth, as the WHO now recognises that without the fulfilment of individual potential, the potential of a community, and even a country cannot be fully met [4]. Lack of health results in a downward spiral that culminates in the inability to utilise or develop inherent skills, resulting in poverty, low standards of living and social inequalities [5]. Those who engage in health-enhancing behaviour simply have access to and make better use of social, educational and employment opportunities [5].

The fulfilment of one's potential allows for what is now termed a 'quality of life', which encompasses many ways of life that have several key features:

- physiological stability
- psychological stability
- the ability to fulfil one's basic needs

- happiness
- self-realisation

The attainment of one's full potential is achieved through adherence to certain principles of living, which may be termed 'a healthy lifestyle' [7]. Self-realisation, or self-fulfilment, is what follows when all the other aspects of health are in place, and one can take up the opportunities that life presents in a state of full physical and mental health and vitality. The study of how one may develop a quality of life and the new health science and research that surround this is termed quality of life medicine [3].

In order to reduce the global economic burden of disease and the extent of human suffering, one needs to ask 'how can we prevent health problems'? [2]. To begin to answer this question, we need to look briefly and simply at the basis of how most diseases arise in our society. But first, we will engage in a little exercise.

Quick Quiz

1. A serious disease is most often the result of:

Answer _____

A. Several lifestyle factors
B. A birth defect
C. A single major problem
D. Factors beyond one's control

2. Quality of life depends on:

Answer _____

A. The opportunities one has
B. The fulfilment of one's potential
C. Attaining good physical health
D. An awareness of spirituality

3. A good definition of health would be:

Answer _____

A. Freedom from pain
B. To be well enough to work
C. To live without needing medicine
D. To be well enough to make the most of oneself

4. One can learn to be happy if:

Answer _____

A. One is well enough to earn a lot of money
B. One achieves one's physical potential by keeping fit
C. One is psychologically and emotionally healthy
D. Life is without stress and one can pay attention to building happiness

5. Health and wealth are:

Answer _____

A. Pretty much the same thing
B. Not the same thing at all
C. Substitutes in that one is as useful as the other
D. Closely connected in that they often go hand in hand

The Characteristics of Communicable and Chronic Diseases

Diseases which are not congenital or due to an accident are generally divided into two types, that of infectious or communicable disease and that of non-communicable or chronic disease [8]. Communicable diseases are characterised by vectors such as:

- Contaminated water
- Airborne bacteria and viruses
- Contaminated or spoilt food
- Parasites
- Direct contact with skin, body fluids or contaminated objects
- Zoonosis (illnesses carried by insects or animals)

Such diseases include:

Tuberculosis	Measles
HIV/AIDS	Meningitis
Infectious Hepatitis	Salmonella
Cholera	Malaria
Norwalk Viruses	Bilharzia

Until 2002 the largest sources of health care problems, the largest numbers of deaths and the major sources of expense were communicable diseases such as HIV/AIDS; Tuberculosis; Dysentery and Hepatitis [2]. The WHO has now realised that there are two sources of health care problem globally: one is the problem of communicable diseases (HIV/AIDS being still the most prevalent) and the other the problem of non-communicable diseases, which in total far outstrip the mortality and morbidity rates of HIV/AIDS as well as the costs [2]. A deadly overlap between communicable and non-communicable diseases and injuries is occurring throughout the developing world, leading to a crisis of priorities for health systems already struggling with inadequate resources.

Non-communicable diseases are those which are generally diseases of lifestyle most often diagnosed in middle age, are not usually curable and may require extensive management [8]. These include:

Cardiovascular disease	Colorectal cancer
Cerebrovascular disease	Obesity
COPD	Type 2 Diabetes Mellitus (T2DM)

The burden of non-communicable diseases is increasing, accounting for nearly half of the global burden of disease (all ages), a 10% increase from estimated levels in 1990. While the proportion of burden from non-communicable diseases in developed countries remains stable at over 80% in adults aged 15 years and over, the proportion in middle-income countries has already exceeded 70%. Surprisingly, almost 50% of the adult disease burden in the high mortality regions of the world is now attributable to non-communicable diseases. Population ageing and changes in the distribution of risk factors have accelerated the epidemic of non-communicable diseases in many developing countries [2]. Under most conditions, non-communicable diseases are preventable by corrective health and lifestyle behaviour. The very term non-communicable, however, is now itself in contention.

Some researchers maintain that the diseases of lifestyle do in fact have vectors; however, these are not the physical or tangible ones of air, water and bacteria but the less tangible social vectors such as social conditions, peer pressure and cultural expectations [8]. The diseases that are carried by such vectors include those of substance abuse, those caused by smoking and alcoholism [8]. Food intake too is subject to cultural and family expectations, extensive marketing campaigns and pressure from the media and peer groups, resulting in a worldwide explosion of obesity and the diseases that relate to it. Such diseases include metabolic syndrome, which results in complex multiple disorders (adult-onset type 2 diabetes, hypertension and increased risk of stroke, cardiovascular disease) some forms of cancer and breathing disorders [8-11].

Learning Together

Activity 1: Allow yourselves 15 minutes for this activity

In small working groups look at the following table and alongside each health problem (disease) tick the most likely categories and causes:

Disease / Problem	Communicable	Chronic / Non-Communicable	Tangible Vector	Social Vector	No Known Cause
Influenza					
Colds					
Alcoholism					
Overweight					
Hypertension					
Migraine					
Stress					
Gastroenteritis					
Asthma					
Eczema					
Meningitis					
STDs					
T2DM					
TB					
Dysentery					

Now you should take 5 minutes to discuss the answers

The Constituents of a Healthy Lifestyle

Many aspects of lifestyle management have recently become part of an international mandate for the improvement of health globally, and the concept is gaining recognition. The World Health Organisation (WHO) identified six main areas of need in health, across the world. These are [12]:

- Hygiene (the control of bacteria and parasites)
- Appropriate and safe fluid intake
- Appropriate dietary guidelines
- Appropriate exercise and self-care
- Substance intake (to include nicotine and alcohol)
- Stress management

These needs can be met for the main part without recourse to pharmaceutical intervention, and many of the goals of good health are within reach of individuals and communities' own self-management. Broadly these can be divided into three categories [3,7,13-16]:

- Attention to physiological aspects of health
- Attention to psychological aspects of health
- Self-expression and awareness of spirituality

Attention to the physiological aspect of health forms the mainstay of lifestyle management. This pertains mainly to the substances we take into our bodies; the physical impact of what we do, as well as our relationship to the elements and our exposure to substances which cause disease.

- Adherence to appropriate dietary guidelines and the consumption of natural unrefined foods;
- Substance intake including those which are safe (clean water and correctly prescribed medication) and the control of those which are unsafe (nicotine, alcohol and recreational drugs);
- Getting adequate amounts of exercise and rest;
- Living a moderately paced lifestyle and
- Avoiding toxins, polluted environments and overexposure to the sun.

Attention to psychological aspects of health:

- Connecting to other people socially;
- Control and management of the impact that stressful situations have on our health;

An awareness of spirituality:

- Being aware of the spiritual aspects of life and
- Having constructive and creative attitudes.

Of these aspects of health, it is mainly the physical impact of nutrition and fitness that has recently come into focus. This is, in part, a good turn of events; however, the focus is not always without commercial bias, and many people have been left confused by an overabundance of conflicting information. To some extent, body image is mediated by culture, with some cultures more concerned about size than others. In multi-ethnic communities, concerns about body mass have been found to be equal in girls of all racial origins; however, the concerns relating to actual dissatisfaction with one's own body shape are not. Research into eating disorders estimated that, at any given time, 35% of teenagers in the UK are dieting, while in fact 7-10% are clinically obese and approximately 1.5% fall into the category of having an eating disorder [17]. Dieting has become a big business, and desperate people often turn to desperate measures and may be the victims of incomplete information and shaky formulas.

Stress is another major lifestyle concern, and the problem is spreading globally. The father of modern stress research, Hans Selye, developed some valuable insights into the nature of stress and its effects on the human physiology. According to Selye, it is not so much the stressor that determines the physiological response but the internal reaction of the individual [18]. Whether they are aware of it or not, most people develop a stress coping mechanism. However, for many, this might be patterns of lifestyle that are ultimately neither conducive to health nor manage the stress or the causes of stress over the long term [19]. The secret of managing stress and moderating the pace of life is to choose mechanisms that are life-enhancing and to build the kind of confidence and ability to cope that is conducive to holistic health. A person's lifestyle is both a major determinant of stress as well as a major determinant of stress management.

We will look at these components of lifestyle in more detail throughout the programme, and we will be learning more about the individual aspects of their management, in depth. We will also be discussing ways in which we can 'cash in' on our new-found knowledge and maximise our potential for health and well-being. Presently, however, we are going to engage in a 'quick quiz' before moving on to our final information section for this learning session.

Quick Quiz

1. Good lifestyle management increases the opportunity for:

Answer _____

A. Health food shop sales
B. Gym membership fees
C. The fulfilment of one's potential
D. Decreasing health care costs

2. Exercise has been proven beneficial:

Answer _____

A. Mainly for participating in sport
B. Mainly for controlling weight
C. For maintaining physical health
D. For maintaining overall physical and mental health

3. Lifestyle management incorporates:

Answer _____

A. Attention to diet and exercise
B. Attention to weight and prevention of obesity
C. Attention to physical and mental health and spirituality
D. Weight control and stress management

4. Appropriately dealing with stress is:

Answer _____

A. Not as important in health as the amount of stress
B. More important in health than the amount of stress
C. Dependant on the source of stress
D. Dependent on whether the stress is physical, mental or emotional

The Importance of Lifestyle Management

We can see that good lifestyle habits are important to health, but how bad is the damage when we do not pay attention to these aspects of health and well-being? Chronic diseases of lifestyle are a group of diseases that share similar risk factors because of exposure over a prolonged period to unhealthy eating habits, lack of exercise, smoking, inappropriate alcohol intake and inappropriate response and control of stress. Such lifestyle habits give rise to hypertension; high levels of inappropriate lipids (fats) in the bloodstream; high blood glucose levels, especially when these occur with insulin resistance, and obesity. Diseases which result from these include stroke, heart disease, tobacco and nutrition-induced cancers, chronic bronchitis, and emphysema [20]. It is estimated that these diseases will increase globally by 77% between 1990 and 2020 mainly in the middle-income sector of the developing world and the social sector of the developed world where there is an insufficient resource to prevent disease [20].

A study that focussed on multiple risk factors in hypertension and CVD found that overweight, alcohol, coffee, sodium and physical inactivity were all risk factors compounded by low intakes of potassium, calcium and magnesium [21]. Previously this was a predominant problem only in developed countries and amongst the wealthy. This is no longer the case, however, and cardiovascular disease is becoming a growing burden in Africa and Asia as well [22]. The main cause of this growing burden of disease is the change in diet in developing countries from an essentially healthy diet, if somewhat restricted in energy, to an intake of food which is more processed, contains more energy but far fewer nutrients [23].

Exercise plays a major role, not only in cardiovascular fitness and prevention of obesity but also in control of stress and alleviation of depression and anxiety [24]. Stress is an area where the impact on health has relatively recently come to light, but some health care professionals feel that it could be the underlying factor responsible for a large proportion of illnesses [6].

Ageing is another problem which has recently had reduced focus since much of the concern has been to reduce child and infant deaths; however, currently, there are 600 million people on the earth who are over 60. Not only will this double by 2025 it is expected to reach 2 billion by 2050. As the ratio of ages in the population changes to one in which older people outnumber those who are healthy and economically active, preventable disorders of ageing will become the new frontier of health care management [2]. Evidence suggests that with an ageing population, the non-communicable or chronic diseases will increase and if the health care systems miss the opportunity to prevent disease in this population. resources will have to be redirected from those which are set aside for child and maternal health. With old-age dependency ratios increasing in virtually all countries of the world, the economic contributions and productive roles of older people will assume greater importance. Supporting people to remain healthy and ensure a good quality of life in their later years is one of the greatest challenges for the health sector in both developed and developing countries [2].

While hereditary disorders and familial tendencies may be factors that one has to learn to live with, the quality of life that results from good management and the lifestyle choices that one makes are entirely under an individual person's control. Nutrition, intake of substances, lifestyle habits, exercise, response to stress and psychological attitudes can be changed, manipulated and managed appropriately. Health and longevity, as well as quality of life medicine, are still areas of ongoing research; however, knowledge surrounding such aspects is developing. We will take an in-depth look at both the positive and negative outcomes of lifestyle practice as we progress through this programme.

Learning Together

Activity 2: Allow yourselves 20 minutes for this activity

In small groups, one person should volunteer an awkward situation that occurred in the last few weeks, in which the outcome was doing something they would have preferred not to do. Choose between the following situations:

1. Going to family or friends for a meal and eating more than you intended – enough to make you feel really uncomfortable
2. Going out with friends intending to have only one drink and having too much
3. Paying for a subscription to a gym, health club, yoga class or keep fit group and not turning up
4. Purchasing exercise equipment, weights or sports clothing which is still unused

Discuss / write down briefly the details and then ask yourself:

Why did I not do what I intended to do in the end?
Was I influenced by another person or people?
Was this influence for the better or worse?
Did I stand up for myself?
Did I argue my point; lose my temper, or use reasoning and common sense to get to my objective?

Each person in the group should try to offer one way of improving the situation, i.e. how things could have been handled better, (this may not necessarily mean getting what the individual wanted).

Now you should take 5 minutes to discuss the answers

Group Discussion

'ACTING UNDER THE INFLUENCE' - THE POWER OF PERSUASION.

Research shows that there are three main factors that predispose a person to either engage in healthy lifestyle management or not. They are predisposing factors (knowledge, beliefs, values and attitudes) enabling factors (access to health education, priorities, commitment and health-related skills) and reinforcing factors (family, friends and mentors)[25]. Reinforcing factors such as the influence of family, friends and mentors, might be the obvious ones when it comes to the power of persuasion. Beliefs and attitudes, however, are formed when one is at an impressionable age, sometimes by family but often because of multiple influences. Commitment, to health and skills building, can also be aided or undermined by people we live, work and socialise with.

Let us discuss a hypothetical situation of being in a coffee shop on a Saturday afternoon with friends or family, or a Saturday night Barbecue (Braaivleis) with a DVD to follow:

- How much of our food intake is determined by choice how much by circumstance and how much by the influence of others?
- Do we drink more alcohol when in the company of others drinking alcohol?
- If we are hosting this occasion, do we make choices on other people's behalf or allow them to make their own choices?
- Is where we sit determined by whether the host or first-person arriving smokes?
- Are we self-conscious about being the only person with a cigarette, alcoholic drink or dessert?
- If we want to consume something 'unhealthy', do we try to persuade others to join us?
- What do we think it would take for us to be able to 'hold our own' and not be under other peoples' influence?

References

1. Merriam-Webster. Merriam-Webster's Medical Dictionary Accessed 2006 26th October. Merriam-Webster Incorporated, 2002.
2. WHO. The World Health Organisation Report 2003 - Shaping the Future. Geneva: World Health Organisation, 2003.
3. Ventegodt S, Kandel I, Merrick J. Principles of Holistic Medicine. Oxford: Trafford Publishing; 2005.
4. WHO. Reducing Risks Promoting Healthy Life. Geneva: World Health Organisation, 2002.
5. Cattell V. Poor people, poor places and poor health: the mediating role of social networks and social capital. Social Science and Medicine. 2001;52:1501-16.
6. Persaud R. The Mind. London: Bantam Press; 2007.
7. Bradley RS. Philosophy of Natural Medicine. In: Pizzorno JE, Murray MT (eds). The Textbook of Natural Medicine. 3rd ed. Volume 1. St Louis: Churchill Livingstone Elsevier, 2006.
8. Ackland M, Choi BCK, Puska P. Rethinking the terms non-communicable disease and chronic disease. British Medical Journal 2003;57(11):838-9.
9. Ando M, Asakura T, Ando S, Simons-Morton BG. Psychosocial factors associated with smoking and drinking among Japanese early adolescent boys and girls: Cross-sectional study. Biomed Central BioPsychoSocial Medicine. 2007;1(13).
10. Bloomgarden ZT. Obesity, Hypertension, and Insulin Resistance. Diabetes Care. 2002;25(11):2088-99.
11. Cannon G (ed). Food, Nutrition and the Prevention of Cancer: a global perspective. Washington DC: World Cancer Research Fund / American Institute for Cancer Research; 1997.
12. WHO. World Health Organisation Report 2004 - Changing History. Geneva: World Health Organisation, 2004.
13. Cranford JA. Stress-buffering or stress-exacerbation? Social support and social undermining as moderators of the relationship between perceived stress and depressive symptoms among married people. Personal Relationships. 2004;11(1):23-40.
14. Grossman P, Niemann L, Schmidt S, Walach H. Mindfulness-based stress reduction and health benefits: A meta-analysis. Journal of Psychosomatic Research. 2003;57:35-43.
15. Oman D, Reed D. Religion and mortality among the community dwelling elderly. American Journal of Public Health. 1998;88:1469-75.
16. Pizzorno L. Spirituality and Healing. In: Pizzorno JE, Murray MT (eds). Textbook of Natural Medicine. Volume 1. St Louis: Churchill Livingstone Elsevier, 2006.
17. Nicholls D, Vilner R. Eating Disorders and Weight Problems. British Medical Journal. 2005;330:950-3.
18. Selye H. The Stress of Life. New York: McGraw Hill; 1978.
19. Murray MT, Pizzorno JE. Stress Management. In: Pizzorno JE, Murray MT (eds). Textbook of Natural Medicine. Volume 1. St Louis: Churchill Livingstone Elsevier, 2006.

20. Murray CJL, Lopez AD. The global burden of disease: a comprehensive assessment of mortality and disability from diseases, injuries and risk factors in 1990 and projected to 2020. In: Bank WHOW (ed): Harvard School of Public Health, 1996.

21. Geleijnse JM, Kok FJ, Grobbee DE. Impact of dietary and lifestyle factors in the prevalence of hypertension in Western populations. European Journal of Public Health. 2004;14(3):235-9.

22. Reddy KS, Yusuf S. Emerging Epidemic of Cardiovascular Disease in Developing Countries. Circulation. 1998;97:596-601.

23. Reddy KS, Katan MB. Diet, nutrition and the prevention of hypertension and cardiovascular diseases. Public Health Nutrition. 2004;71(A)(Supplement 1):167-86.

24. Lutack B, Bongiorno PB. The Exercise Prescription. In: Pizzorno JE, Murray MT (eds). Textbook of Natural Medicine. 3rd ed. Volume 1. St Louis: Churchill Livingstone Elsevier, 2006.

25. Johnson PH, Kittleson MJ. A Qualitative Exploration of Health Behaviours and the Associated Factors among University Students from Different Cultures. The International Electronic Journal of Health Education. Volume 6, 2003:14-25.

LEARNING SESSION TWO: THE IMPORTANCE OF NUTRITION AND THE ESSENTIAL BUILDING BLOCKS OF A GOOD DIET

Introduction

Nutrition is currently a hot topic and has been the subject of TV programmes, radio talks, chat shows and reality TV programmes. Nutrition has hit the media in magazine articles, books and celebrity diets; however, how much do we really know and how do we know that what we are being told is right or not? There is plenty of information on the internet and in popular fad diet books but what we do with it and how we wade through it all to find out what we can apply and how requires a little guidance.

This session looks at the essential nutrients that we require for good health. These fall into two groups: the macronutrients, being carbohydrates, fats and proteins, and the micronutrients, being vitamins and minerals. We look at the best forms of macronutrients, and the food sources of the types of carbohydrates and fats and proteins that benefit us the most. This will be followed by our first learning together session.

Micronutrients are important, and we look at just how many are essential and the possible consequences of having insufficient of these tiny but vital substances. Nutritional imbalance plays a major role in disease, and we finally highlight how good nutrition can be a major preventative measure against future ill-health. Our second learning together session is followed by our discussion for the day ' Malnutrition in Modern Societies' are we becoming overfed but undernourished?

Ice-Breaker Quiz

Let us see how much you know already about the subject of food and nutrition. Can you separate the myths from the facts?   **Myth / Fact**

1. Cream and butter contain as much protein as milk and cheese.   _____

2. Vitamins and minerals are useless if they are cooked they only count if they are eaten raw.   _____

3. Fibre is essential to health but is often missing from processed foods.   _____

4. One good meal per day is enough; a healthy adult does not need to eat more than this.   _____

5. Children require less food and fewer nutrients than adults.   _____

6. Older people require more nutrients such as vitamins and minerals but possibly fewer calories than younger adults.   _____

7. The human body contains more water than any other substance, which is why drinking water is important.   _____

8. Digesting food requires water, so if one is eating less one needs to drink less.   _____

9. Protein is where we get most of our energy from, and we should ideally eat as much as we can afford to.   _____

10. Fruits and vegetables are our biggest sources of vitamins and many necessary minerals.   _____

Ice-Breaker Quiz

The Importance of Nutrition in a Lifestyle Programme

Food and drink are the main items we take in to sustain ourselves. In this respect, nutrition forms one of the major cornerstones of health (the others being hygiene, exercise and rest). The quality of nutrition determines, in many respects, the quality of our health and ultimately the quality of our life [1]. Nutrition is, in addition, one of the major mediators of health that is totally under our own control and not dependant on physical ability, has little to do with finance and can be adequate, even with minimal resources, if we have the underlying information with which to make appropriate choices.

Under-nutrition is defined as insufficient nutrients due to inadequate food intake or inadequate assimilation of food (due to illness or gastrointestinal disorders), whereas malnutrition is due to an unbalanced intake of nutrients [2]. These are not necessarily mutually exclusive. That means that although one can be undernourished, one may or may not have the correct balance of nutrients. In the case of malnutrition, one may be undernourished as well, and the problem is that one is receiving both too little food and too little variety of foods. Traditionally we associate these two disorders with one another, and these two terms have sometimes been used interchangeably.

Increasingly in modern times and in developed countries, one finds that there is malnutrition that is simply due to imbalances in food intake and not due to either undernutrition or necessarily shortages of food, poverty or gastrointestinal problems. Causes of this type of malnutrition are that either too little variety is eaten, or too much food with low nutritional value is consumed. This occurs, for instance, when people eat chips (fries) with almost every meal or centre each main meal on meat and potatoes. They have too many calories (which we will come to later) and too few essential nutrients, a scenario which leads to many chronic disorders over the long term.

The science of nutrition has changed over the last few years, and where once a balanced diet was one where one ate adequately enough to avoid nutrient deficiencies, we are now at the stage where good nutrition means consuming an optimum diet for promoting health as well as reducing the risk of diet-related disorders. At the turn of the last century, scientists began to embrace the use of optimum nutrition which focuses on optimising the quality of the diet, not only in terms of nutritional content but also in terms of non-nutrients as well as other food properties that favour the maintenance and enhancement of health [3]. The WHO report on the prevention of chronic diseases highlighted lifestyle related disorders that were strongly linked to long-term nutritional imbalance. The report also adopted an individualistic approach which encourages each person to make individual and sensible dietary choices [4].

There have been more advances in public health made by the reduction of risk than by the application of medication for illness, a fact which is often overlooked in the fight against disease

5. The promotion of laws regarding health and safety in the workplace, in hospitals and on the roads, as well as public water supplies, and the handling of food have contributed in some respects to decreases in some types of diseases and certain causes of death. Too many of us are living dangerously, however, as a result of making the wrong lifestyle choices, particularly with respect to our intake of food [5].

An essential nutrient is one which is necessary for our survival. The term 'essential' means two things, firstly that we cannot survive for any meaningful length of time without problems if we do not have this nutrient and secondly, that we cannot manufacture it ourselves. Essential nutrients are those that we must take in from the outside, through foods and fluids in our diet. Essential nutrients are found in all unprocessed unrefined foods, and they come in two forms; those that we require in bulk are called the *macronutrients*, and those that we require in smaller amounts are termed *micronutrients*.

All organotrophic organisms (trophe is the Greek word for food) ultimately obtain their energy from the sun through a process called *photosynthesis*. Plants pick up carbon dioxide (CO_2) from the air and water (H_2O) from the soil and combine these to form carbon bonds in the molecules that make up the plant's tissue. Plants convert energy from light into chemical energy, which is stored within the carbon bonds [6].

Carbohydrate is a chemical name for hydrate (water) of carbon [7]. Plants also incorporate inorganic nitrogen from nitrogen-fixing bacteria to form *amino acids*, which are the building blocks of proteins. Animals (and humans) eat the plants and convert the amino acids to the proteins that they require for growth and repair [6]. Although plants have the ability to pick up carbon dioxide from the air and water from the ground, animals do not; hence all of their carbohydrates have to be eaten in the form of plants (or from the intestines of animals that they kill for food)[7]. Carbohydrates, lipids and proteins form the basis of what we eat, the macronutrients. These are the nutrients we need a lot of, and from where we obtain all our energy. Within these, the micronutrients are found, which we require in smaller amounts. The amount and absorbability by the body of these micronutrients depend heavily on the overall quality of the food containing them. Low quality and highly processed food may translate into inadequate micronutrients. Although required in small amounts, the absence of some of these contributes to diseases such as hypertension, increasing the risk of stroke and osteoporosis, which increases the risk of fractures.

One of the most effective tools of preventative medicine is nutrition education and intervention. Changing the eating habits of a group of people, would cut the figures for heart disease, diabetes and some of the preventable cancers along with the misery that comes with them. Many chronic diseases are not only preventable but, if caught in time, can be dealt with solely with a change in diet. Unfortunately, it sometimes takes a crisis in a person's life for them to begin looking at ways to help themselves out of a chronic ill-health problem and to look at ways to prevent further degeneration [8].

Quick Quiz

Below are several measures that may be viewed either as bad lifestyle choices, or they may prevent disease, unnecessary deaths and accidents, and promote health. Using coloured pencils or pens place a circle around the words or phrases that you think are the ones being asked for:

1. Circle in red the laws that prevent accidents and deaths
2. Circle in green the lifestyle choices that build health and well-being
3. Circle in blue the factors that can be viewed as lifestyle choices that endanger health
4. Circle in yellow the factors that can reduce disease but which you might require skills to accomplish or could not accomplish on your own

speed limits on roads   cigarette smoking   eating fresh fruit

reduction in air pollution   wearing seatbelts in cars

drinking alcohol,   a daily walk   handrails on stairs

fire alarm systems   clean and safe drinking water

growing your own vegetables   adequate sleep

food shopping for quality   overeating

skipping breakfast   matching food intake
to requirements

Quantity and Quality of Carbohydrates and Lipids (fats)

Carbohydrates

Carbohydrates can be classified as simple carbohydrates such as:

- Monosaccharides (single sugars) such as glucose and fructose
- Disaccharides (double sugars) and oligosaccharides (a few sugars) such as sucrose, lactose and maltose

Or complex carbohydrates:

- Polysaccharides (many sugars) such as starches
- non-digestible polymers (fibres, pectins and gums) sometimes known as non-starch polysaccharides or NSP.

The chemical formula for glucose is $C_6H_{12}O_6$. A glucose molecule plus a fructose molecule together make sucrose, the simple sugar we know in crystalline form as table sugar. Many glucose molecules linked together form chains of molecules to become starch, which is harder to break down and takes longer to digest. The structure of plant carbohydrates account for their variation in physiological properties and is linked to their function. As a general rule, the simpler the carbohydrate molecule, the sweeter the substance and the more easily and quickly it is broken down by the body and absorbed [6] Glucose is oxidised in the body to give energy and heat:

$$C_6H_{12}O_6 + 6O_2 \longrightarrow 6CO_2 + 6H_2O + Energy + Heat$$

Glucose   Carbon Dioxide   Water

Glucose is the most widely distributed sugar in nature, although it is usually consumed in the form of starches and cellulose. Glucose linked with fructose forms sucrose and makes up a large fraction of the content of fruits and vegetables, alongside some of the non-digestible starches. Fructose is the sweetest of all the monosaccharides, and between 1% and 7% fructose can be found in most fruits. As fruit ripens, enzymes split the sucrose molecules into glucose and fructose, which results in a sweeter taste. Fructose makes up about 3% of vegetables and 40% of honey. Galactose is another simple sugar but hardly found in nature except for breast milk, together with glucose it forms the basis of lactose, the disaccharide found in dairy products, and which comprises about 4.5% of milk [6]. Disaccharides are broken down first to split them into monosaccharides. This requires the enzymes invertase (to split sucrose), maltase (to split maltose) and lactase (to split lactose). The insufficiency of the latter is sometimes a problem which occurs predominantly in persons of Asian and Central African origin and about 10% of Europeans [6].

Complex carbohydrates in the form of both digestible and non-digestible starches are broken down more slowly, maintaining a steady flow of glucose and energy. The non-digestible portion of the carbohydrate (NSP) or fibre, slows down the absorption and provides a fermentable base for the production of health-enhancing 'friendly' bacteria in the large intestines [6].

Plants store carbohydrates as starch by linking chains of glucose into a complex granular structure. The more complex carbohydrate the plant makes during photosynthesis, the greater the rate of starch formation. Complex carbohydrates are the main source of energy in most countries in the world and the metabolically 'preferred' source of energy for the body. In most parts of the developing world 50-80% of the total energy taken in comes from carbohydrate-rich foods, a proportion of carbohydrate that has kept humans from extinction and allowed it to grow and flourish for many thousands of years. However, with economic development, the proportion of energy taken in from carbohydrate foods drops to 40-50% of the total energy intake, of which an increasing amount comes from refined simple sugars. As less unrefined and complex starch is consumed, the amount of NSP in the diet also decreases [6].

Because the structure is complex, raw starch cannot be broken down and requires moist cooking which causes the cells containing the starch molecules to swell and gelatinise, rupturing the cell walls and making it more digestible. Some starch remains (resistant starch) yielding limited amounts of glucose for absorption. Complex carbohydrates (including starch) release glucose slowly and is therefore useful in sustaining energy over a longer period of time [6].

A growing body of evidence now suggests that dietary carbohydrates, especially NSP, have a significant impact on human physiology. Specific carbohydrates modulate whole-body energy processes and, in addition, affect certain disease processes. Carbohydrates in all forms are broken down by enzymes which split the glycosidic links holding the molecules of monosaccharides together. The fewer the glycosidic linkages, the quicker the process, which is why monosaccharides, which do not require enzymatic action, and disaccharides with only one link to break down are absorbed from the digestive system and enter the bloodstream very quickly. This is especially the case in the absence of dietary fibre.

The net result of such a process is that simple carbohydrates and foods containing predominantly monosaccharides and disaccharides are broken down and released into the bloodstream in a short amount of time. This elevates the blood glucose level, which in turn, triggers the pancreas into releasing insulin. Insulin is a hormone that carries the glucose molecule across the cell wall, thus providing some of the 'starter material' for the production of energy within the body's cells [6]. The brain is the most important recipient of glucose from the blood, without a steady and constant stream of glucose crossing the blood-brain barrier the brain cannot function adequately [6]. Periodic surges in blood glucose trigger insulin release which carries the glucose into the cells, however, with constant 'priming' for insulin release the pancreas can become oversensitive, releasing too much insulin too quickly, resulting in dips in the level of glucose below the amount necessary for optimum brain function. This accounts for a problem known as 'reactive' hypoglycaemia, the symptoms of which include sudden hunger, cravings for sweets, anxiety, shakiness, cold sweats, pallor, disorientation or confusion [9].

More complex carbohydrates, however, require a longer chemical process of splitting the numerous glycosidic links, releasing the individual molecules much more slowly into the system. In addition, unrefined complex carbohydrates are more likely to contain significant levels of micronutrients and are bound together with significant amounts of NSP as well as some small amounts of dietary fats, thus allowing for a longer, slower process of digestion and absorption [6]. The benefit of such foods is that when one consumes these, one feels more satisfied and sustains a steady energy level for longer [6].

The trick with carbohydrate consumption is not to restrict carbohydrates *per se* as this can lead to many other problems, including those resulting from lack of fibre and insufficient anti-oxidant nutrients. There is a good amount of evidence to support the value of eating plenty of carbohydrates in the form of fresh fruits and vegetables, whole grains and pulses to reduce our risk of diseases such as cancer [10], hypertension and stroke, [11] cardiac heart disease [12] and the problems inherent in ageing [13] including macular degeneration which is a leading cause of blindness in older people [14]. The effects of refining carbohydrates, however, remove much of the fibre and many of the B-complex vitamins and minerals. This has the effect of speeding up the time it takes to break the glycosidic links and facilitate absorption as well as lowering the nutritional content of the food item overall [10]. Unrefined carbohydrate-rich foods have enormous benefits if we choose them wisely, including:

- Regulating blood glucose levels and providing a steady, stable stream of energy to the body's cells including those in the brain
- Providing adequate amounts of dietary fibre which regulates fat absorption and controls the amount of undesirable fats absorbed into the bloodstream
- Providing most of our water-soluble and many of our fat-soluble vitamins
- Providing our best sources of many essential minerals

Lipids

Lipid is the chemical name for a group of compounds which includes fats, oils and fat-related substances such as cholesterol and lecithin. Fats and lipids too have a simple structure of carbon, hydrogen and oxygen atoms and, like carbohydrates, their properties and functions in the body are also linked closely to their structure. Lipids are compounds that frequently occur in nature and are an important part of the plant, animal and microbial membranes. The definition of a lipid is based on its solubility. While carbohydrates are soluble in water, lipids are only marginally soluble in water (at best) and are soluble in organic solvents such as acetone and chloroform. Fats and oils are typical lipids in terms of their solubility [15].

Lipids are the building blocks of fats found in both plant and animal-derived foods. Unlike carbohydrates, these are smaller structures, are very dense and contain 2.25 (two and a quarter) times the energy of carbohydrate. Human beings store fat as energy for future use in times of famine. There are two types of fat in the human body; the most important is *structural fat* (known as 'brown fat') which helps to keep the organs in place and protect the nerves from shock and damage. This type of fat contributes to subcutaneous fat, which acts as insulation, preserving and regulating body temperature. The second type is *adipose tissue* or stored fat. Dietary fats, found in fish, seeds, nuts, whole grains, avocado pears and olives are essential for the digestion, absorption, and transport of fat-soluble vitamins [16]. There are three major groups of lipids that we are most concerned with in respect of nutrition are:

> Fatty acids
> Triglycerides
> Phospholipids

Fatty acids are those that are essential as far as food intake is concerned as the body makes triglycerides and phospholipids from the fatty acids, all of which are found in foods. They may be either saturated or unsaturated Saturated fats are found in animal-derived products, but it is the unsaturated fats (usually referred to as oils) found in cold water fish and vegetable products that are essential. If all the available bonds are used up (i.e. there is no extra space for another atom or molecule to attach itself), then the fat is said to be 'saturated'. Unsaturated fats have some double bonds between their carbon atoms, are liquid at room temperature and are often characterised by the location of these double bonds (characterised by the Greek letter 'ẃ' – omega) which gives them different chemical properties. A monounsaturated fatty acid has a single, double bond, and polyunsaturated fatty acids have two or more double bonds [15]. The three essential fatty acids are [16]:

- Oleic Acid   ẃ 9 $C_{18}H_{34}O_2$ 1 double bond
  - found in olives, canola seeds, and linseeds
- Linoleic Acid   ẃ 6 $C_{18}H_{32}O_2$ 2 double bonds
  - found in most nuts, seeds, grains, avocado pears, soy, peanuts and linseeds
- Alpha Linolenic Acid ẃ 3 $C_{18}H_{30}O_2$ 3 double bonds
  - found in fish (salmon, sardines, pilchards, mackerel), walnuts, and linseeds

Lipids constitute just over a third (34%) of the energy intake of the average diet and can store energy in the form of fats in adipocytes, the cells that form adipose tissue. The ability to store and use large amounts of fats originally enabled humans to survive without food for weeks, or even months, during periods of drought, cold and famine. This ability contributed to the survival of early humans [6].

Lipids have many vital functions in the body. They account for 15% of the normal body weight of men and 20% of the normal body weight of women. At least half of this is stored under the skin as adipose tissue the rest provides insulation, cushions vital organs, and carries nutrients in the blood. Adipose tissue fat can be burned for energy provided carbohydrate is present.

Fat as an energy source is very concentrated, providing nine calories per gram as against carbohydrate and protein, which provide four calories per gram. Lipids are present in cell membranes and transport vitamins A,D,E, and K through the body. Deficiency of essential linoleic acid causes red and scaly skin, stunted growth in children, dehydration and infections [6]. Fats in the form of sterols (or cholesterol) are also essential for Production of steroids and hormones in the body and the structure of the walls of individual cells in the body [6].

Triglycerides

Fatty acids are rarely found 'free' in nature; biologic organisms link three fatty acids to a molecule of glycerol to form a triglyceride. Most lipids in foods (more than 95%) and in the body are in the form of triglycerides. When we are talking about fat, either in food or in the body, we really are talking about triglycerides. Fatty acids linked to glycerol are usually neutral and non-reactive, they can be safely transported in the blood and stored in fat cells (adipose tissue) without doing any damage [6].

Phospholipids

Phospholipids are triglycerides that contain a phosphate molecule, one end and at the other end a nitrogen-containing molecule (usually choline, serine or inositol). The phosphate-containing portion of this molecule forms hydrogen bonds with water, thus making the whole phospholipid more soluble in water and giving it the ability to carry the fat portions into the digestive juices, thus enabling the digestion and absorption of fats [6].

A very important phospholipid is phosphatidylcholine (commonly known as lecithin), which is used to transport fats and cholesterol in the body. Lecithin is essential to the body, as it is a component of cell membranes and has been found in the memory cells of the brain. It can be manufactured in the liver. Lecithin acts as a fat emulsifier, keeping it in solution in the blood and in other parts of the body. Lecithin is widely distributed in the food chain, the best sources being egg yolks, soybeans, peanuts, legumes and spinach [6].

Cholesterol

Cholesterol is probably the best-known fat related compound. It belongs to a class of lipid substances called sterols. It is obtained from certain foods, those containing saturated and animal fats, however, the body also manufactures cholesterol from adipose fat, sugars, and amino acids consumed in excess, or not needed by the body's cells [6]. Cholesterol is widely distributed in our body's cells and is a vital component of the cell membrane. It is also found in large amounts of the brain and nerve tissue, and it forms the steroid base of all the sex hormones. A cholesterol derivative which lies under the surface of the skin cells reacts to sunlight on the skin and forms vitamin D, which carries bone-building minerals from the blood to the bone cells. Cholesterol is also used in making bile acids that function in the digestion of fats [6]. Cholesterol in food is found in organ meats, eggs, dairy products, meat, poultry, fish and shellfish [6].

Lipoproteins

Fat is the most energy dense constituent of the diet, and its contribution to dietary energy rises with industrialisation and urbanisation of the population. Oils and fats are present in most foods to a greater or lesser extent; however, meat from domesticated animals has a high-fat content as have many manufactured foods. In addition, oils and fats are often added at the table [10]. Also, food often contains a mixture of both saturated and unsaturated triglycerides and phospholipids, which bind to a greater or lesser degree with proteins. In this form, we refer to them as lipoproteins. It is in the form of lipoproteins that fats are carried around in the blood. High-density lipoproteins (HDL) contain more proteins and fewer triglycerides and cholesterol and aid in clearing the less good fats from the system. Low-density lipoproteins (LDL) arise out of saturated fats and trans-fatty acids from processed foods and carry the greater portion of cholesterol in the blood. It is LDLs that are responsible for the damage to the lining of the blood vessels [17]. In the fight against cardiac disease and cancer, it has been found to be overall beneficial to have more HDL than LDL in the blood [10,17].

The ideal ratio of fats

Some fats are useful, some are less useful, and some are not useful at all. It has been postulated that humans evolved by consuming a diet lower in saturated fat and higher in ώ3 fatty acids than is consumed today. Ancient peoples either lived by the oceans and consumed fish and fruits or lived inland and consumed a diet far higher in plant foods than is currently consumed [18]. Man's original diet is thought to have been richer in marine and plant sources of ώ3 fats and lower in ώ6 fats resulting in a ratio of 1:1 ώ3: ώ6. In contrast, the modern diet is richer in ώ6 from both animal protein and oils extracted from grains such as corn and safflower oils [6]. The current recommendation is that the ώ6:ώ3 ratio should be between 2:1 and 3:1, which is approximately four times lower than the current average intake of ώ6 fatty acids [6]. Also ώ9 fats, as in olive oil, are to be taken into consideration as some benefit has been shown from a diet which features olive oil as opposed to more saturated oils or refined grain extracted oils [12] [11]. Most dietary intake as previously stated is far higher in ώ6 fats, this is partly because such fats are inherent anyway in the grains we consume, and in many breakfast cereals that contain nuts and seeds. To balance this, one should aim to take in any additional fats in the form of ώ3 or ώ9 where possible.

Quick Quiz

Below are several carbohydrate and lipid-containing foods; using coloured pencils or pens place a circle around the words or phrases that you think are the ones being asked for:

1. Circle in red the food items comprised mainly of simple carbohydrates
2. Circle in green the food items that contain saturated fatty acids
3. Circle in blue the food items containing complex carbohydrates
4. Circle in yellow the foods containing unsaturated essential fatty acids

boiled sweets   pork chops   sweet potatoes

candy floss   broccoli   poached egg

molasses   sardines   avocado pear

ham and cheese omelette   baked potato with ratatouille

olives   roast rack of lamb   apricot jam

peanut butter   macaroni with mushrooms and beans

fudge   grilled chicken wings   cashew nuts   multigrain bagel

The Importance of Protein: What it is and What it does

Proteins are built from chains of amino acids. Amino acids are carbohydrates with an amino group added (NH_2 – containing nitrogen). There are 20 amino acids required by humans, which fall into two groups; essential and non-essential. Essential ones are those that humans cannot make, and we have no option but to obtain them from our diet. The essential amino acids are [6]:

Phenylalanine	P
Valine	v
Threonine	T
Tryptophan	T
Isoleucine	I
Methionine	M
Histidine	H
Arginine	A
Lysine	L
Leucine	L

Everything that lives, (plants, trees, flowers, insects and animals and of course human beings) are built on proteins. Other than water, proteins are the chief constituents of the human body. The word Protein is derived from the Greek word *proteios,* which means 'of first importance' [7]. Whereas plant structures are primarily composed of carbohydrates, the structures of animals and humans are built on proteins [6]. Proteins function in the body in the building of new cells, the maintenance of existing cells and the replacement of old cells. Proteins (as hormones) regulate metabolic processes, and (as enzymes) catalyse metabolic processes; they transport oxygen in the blood (as haemoglobin) and (as antibodies) defend the body against infection. Proteins (as nerves) transmit impulses and allow us to move by contracting our muscles. Proteins are components of skin, hair, nails and all our internal supporting tissue [7]. Another very important role of proteins is in helping to maintain the water balance in our bodies [6]. In addition, hormones, blood cells and other body chemicals also have a protein base, and the DNA that makes up the core master centre of the nucleus of our cells and our genetic characteristics are made up from the amino acids that form the building blocks of proteins [6].

Protein in muscles and body tissues is in a state of constant turnover, as tissue protein is degraded, nitrogen is excreted in the urine, and new protein is required daily in order to maintain the body in a stable state [6]. Infection, traumatic injury, pregnancy and rapid growth in infancy and early childhood increase the requirement for protein and amino acid synthesis. If this is not met, the body goes into a negative nitrogen balance, where more nitrogen is excreted than is being taken in. This, in turn, results in the body breaking down muscle tissue in order to facilitate essential repair and maintenance of the immune system, combat infection and prevent sepsis [6].

The problem of negative nitrogen balance and accompanying muscle wasting and lack of tissue repair and maintenance is nowhere more apparent than in those who suffer from anorexia and other eating disorders [12]. Muscle mass is often equated with the circulating amino acid pool as similar quantities of muscle are destroyed and rebuilt every day. Increasing the muscle mass with resistance exercises increases the body's nitrogen turnover and its requirements, however, this also enhances the physical ability of the body to metabolise protein as well as carbohydrate [19].

Although individuals will have their own unique requirements for proteins, overall, the total protein recommendation for the average adult is 0.8 grams per kg of body weight. The World Health Organisation (WHO) has issued a mandate that the minimum protein intake for an adult should be 23 grams [20]. Protein is found in most foods, even if it is in only small amounts. As plants too require amino acids, there will be proteins in both plant and animal sources of foods. In general, protein makes up [10]:

- 20-36% of the weight of most pulses
- 8-25% of nuts and seeds
- 8-16% of whole grains
- 10-20% of meat and fish
- 15% of eggs
- 3-4% of milk
- 1-3% of vegetables

There is little, if any, difference between the quality of protein of animal origin and that of plant origin when the latter includes both grains and pulses. Plant protein sources provide 65% of the world food supply of edible protein of which cereals comprise 47% and pulses nuts and seeds approximately 8%. Intakes of plant protein vary little; however, intakes of animal sources of protein increases with economic prosperity [10].

The WHO recognised the way of evaluating how useful a particular food is in terms of meeting our protein requirements is its 'protein digestibility corrected amino acid score (PDCAAS). Proteins that provide amino acids equal to or more than requirements receive a score of 1 (or 100%). A food with a score of 1 will meet the total protein needs of a human being during periods of growth when consumed as a sole source of protein at the minimum required rate (0.8 g / kg for adults)[6,20,21]. Some examples of the PDCAAS scores of commonly consumed foods are:

Yoghurt	1	Whole grain rye	0.68
Egg	1	Oats	0.57

Milk or cheese	1	Whole wheat	0.54
Soy	1	Lentils	0.52
Lean beef	0.92	Peanuts	0.52
Peas	0.73	Brown Rice	0.47
Kidney beans	0.68	Corn	0.42

Closely related species of plants tend to make proteins of a similar amino acid profile; however, very different species tend to contain a different amino acid profile. Food combinations that provide all the required amino acids giving a full PDCAAS score of 1 include [6]:

Combinations	Examples
Whole grains and legumes (pulses)	Lentil biryani
	Gnushu (corn and beans)
	Bean soup and rye bread
	Bean burritos
	Dhal and rice
	Beans on whole wheat toast
	Peanut butter sandwich
Legumes (pulses) and seeds	Hummus with tahini
	Falafel
	Lentil and sesame pâté
Whole grains and dairy	Whole grain pasta and fromage frais
	Müsli and yoghurt

Learning Together

Activity 2.1 Allow yourselves 15 minutes for this activity

From what you now know about carbohydrates, fats and proteins: What do you think are the main differences between the following two meals?

A. White rice with sweetened carrots and peas served with meatballs and ketchup
B. Wholegrain brown rice cooked with lentils, almonds and spices served with eggplant (aubergines) and squash in a tomato-based sauce

Which meal do you think contains more utilisable protein?
Which meal do you think will satisfy you for longer?
Why do you think this is so?

Now you should take 5 minutes to discuss the answers

The Micronutrients: Great Things from Small Packages!

The *micronutrients* are those that are essential to our health and well-being, but we need them in small amounts. They are found within the carbohydrate, lipid and protein-rich foods that produce energy. While the basic functions of the macronutrients are to produce energy for both immediate use and storage and to build and repair body tissues, micronutrients function at the cellular level. That is, they come into our systems via food, which is broken down and digested in the stomach and small intestines, from where the micronutrients are extracted and absorbed into the bloodstream to circulate around the body and 'feed' the individual cells which make up the tissues. Micronutrients consist of *vitamins, minerals, phytonutrients and fibre*. Here we will briefly introduce them.

Vitamins

It was the discovery of vitamins that led to the birth of the science that we now know as nutrition. Vitamins, which are essential micronutrients, have the following criteria [22]:

- They are organic compounds (contain carbon), but distinct from the macronutrients (carbohydrates, lipids and proteins).
- They are natural components of unprocessed foods, present usually in minute amounts.
- They are not synthesised in the body in any amount that would be considered adequate to meet normal physiological needs – they are therefore essential.
- Insufficiency of these substances causes a specific deficiency syndrome that adversely affects one's health.

There are eighteen vitamins and vitamin-like substances that we require as humans for health [22]. There are two types of vitamins, those that are fat soluble and those that are water soluble. The fat-soluble vitamins are passively absorbed from food – that is they need a little help and require to be transported with a dietary lipid. They tend to be found in the lipid portions of the cellular component of the food. Fat-soluble vitamins can be stored in the body to a certain extent, and therefore, the body can sustain itself for a short time if these are not taken in daily. The fat-soluble vitamins are [22]:

- Vitamin A - Retinol, retinal, retinoic acid
- Vitamin E - α-tocopherol
- Vitamin D - Cholecalciferol
- Vitamin K - Phylloquinone, menaquinone, menadione

Vitamins A and E work together as antioxidants to protect the integrity of the cell membrane. Vitamins D and K work together to build healthy bones

Vitamin A deficiency is the most prevalent cause of blindness the world over. It is estimated that in developing countries, 250 million children are at risk and between 250,000 and 500,000 cases of vitamin A deficiency-related blindness occurs annually. The first sign of vitamin A deficiency occurs as 'night blindness', the inability to adjust to the dark, followed by skin anomalies, such as dry, bumpy skin, first noticed on the backs of the upper arms. Further deficiencies result in an impaired immune function [22].

Vitamin A related substances known as carotenoids (including beta-carotene) represent the most widespread group of naturally occurring pigments in nature. They are a highly coloured (red and yellow) group of fat-soluble compounds. More than 600 have been discovered, but only about 30-50 are believed to have any vitamin A related activity [22]. The best sources of vitamin A and Beta-carotene are contained in the red and orange pigments of food; sometimes this colouring is overlaid with chlorophyll giving the foods a dark green colour. In general, foods of animal origin contain vitamin A and those of vegetable origin beta-carotene [22].

The water-soluble vitamins are absorbed both by passive and active mechanisms and may be transported by carriers or absorbed directly from the intestines into the bloodstream. They are found in the aqueous (or watery) parts of the cells of foods. Unlike fat-soluble vitamins, water-soluble vitamins cannot be stored by the body and, once absorbed, metabolised and used; any excess is flushed out in the urine. This means that they need to be taken in on a daily basis [22] these are [22]:

- Vitamin C   - Ascorbic Acid
- Vitamin B Complex
    - B1   - Thiamin
    - B2   - Riboflavin
    - B3   - Niacin
    - B5   - Pantothenic Acid
    - B6   - Pyridoxine
    - -   - Folate
    - B12   - Cobalamin
    - -   - Biotin

Vitamin C is responsible mainly for the integrity of the blood vessels, skin and the immune system but has many other functions as well. The B-complex vitamins are important in nerve function and conduction of messages along the neural pathway as well as having other important metabolic functions connected with the generation of energy within the cells [22].

Vitamins are obtained mainly from fresh vegetables and fruits, as well as whole grains, pulses, nuts, seeds, and eggs. Other vitamin-like substances that are not strictly vitamins but work together with vitamins and have what is termed vitamin-like behaviour in the body include the substances Choline; Carnitine; myo-Inositol; and the Ubiquinones and Bioflavonoids . These substances occur naturally in most foods, alongside the other vitamins and as long as your diet has a good variety of whole foods, you will most likely not be deficient in these micronutrients [22].

Minerals

The minerals are a large class of micronutrients, most of which are essential. They are found in unprocessed foods and exist in the body, mainly in the *ionic* (elemental) state. Although we do not need these in any large amounts as we do the bulk nutrients, there are some minerals that we require in a measurable amount on a daily basis, 100 mg or more (examples are magnesium and calcium) which are termed *macrominerals* and some for which the requirement is very small indeed, this being 15 mg or less (such as iron and zinc), known as *trace elements*. Recently the term *'ultra-trace elements'* has been used to describe those minerals that we require in microgram (μg) quantities each day, (such as selenium and chromium) [23].

Minerals have many essential functions in the body, including serving as ions dissolved in water which keep the 'electrical flow' of the body moving. This is essential for heart and muscle function, as well as the functioning of the nervous system. In addition, minerals maintain the balance of water inside and outside of the body's cells, and the correct acidic balance of the body. Minerals form components of the body's cells, which is especially vital in the bone structure and, in addition, maintain the activities of enzyme systems [23].

The 18 essential minerals that we require are [23]:

Calcium	Ca	Fluorine	Fl
Phosphorous	P	Copper	Cu
Magnesium	Mg	Iodine	I
Sodium	Na	Selenium	Se
Potassium	K	Manganese	Mn
Chloride	Cl	Chromium	Ch
Sulphur	S	Molybdenum	Mo
Iron	Fe	Boron	Bo
Zinc	Zn	Cobalt	Co

Research into how the body utilises minerals and our requirements for minerals has lagged a little behind the knowledge we have acquired about the vitamins. Although we may not know exactly how much we need of the ultra-trace elements on a daily basis for good health, we have begun to recognise that they are nevertheless necessary and should not be left out [23]. One ongoing problem with minerals is that plant food, supposedly rich in certain minerals, may not contain as much as we would expect if grown in poor quality soil. This is especially bad in countries where poor farming methods are used or where farmers do not have the money to buy good quality fertiliser or the knowledge of good use of their land. This could mean that in poor communities where nutrition is already compromised, things might be made worse when the food that is consumed has less than the expected quantities of nutrients.

Although not strictly speaking individual nutrients, such as vitamins or minerals, both fibre and phytonutrients have come under the spotlight more due to the adverse effects of their absence from the diet as much as due to their presence.

Dietary fibre

Dietary fibre is a component of carbohydrates. While the component of starch comes from the inside of the plant, fibre comes mainly from the structural walls. The cellular structure is slightly different from that of starches. Fibre takes a number of forms, each of which has different properties [24]:

- Cellulose
- Hemicellulose
- Pectins
- Gums

Fibre nevertheless has several essential functions in the gastrointestinal system, including [24]:

- Regulation of the absorption of sugars
- Regulation of the absorption of fats
- Encouraging adequate and regular peristalsis in the gastrointestinal tract

Many nutritional scientists blame may diseases that previously did not exist and are which are prevalent in Westernised societies on the insufficiency of fibre in the diet. Some chronic degenerative diseases can be avoided by increasing dietary fibre and the consumption of unrefined plant foods as part of ones nutritional and lifestyle improvement plan [25] [26].

Phytonutrients

Phytonutrients are small amounts of substances found in herbs, spices and other food-related items, but they are not complete foods. They may have special health-enhancing properties over and above the benefits of the intake of macro-nutrients and baseline amounts of micro-nutrients. There can be two reasons for this:

- The item has a particularly high content of one or more micro-nutrients which have been found beneficial in mitigating or preventing a specific disorder.
- The food has a phytochemical component which has medicinal properties.

Phytonutrients are often used traditionally and can be incorporated easily into cooking, examples being garlic, cayenne pepper, ginger and turmeric. Many herbal teas also contain nutritional substances and have medicinal properties, such as peppermint, rooibos (red bush) and green tea.

Quick Quiz

Given below are certain properties that pertain to foods or components of foods, using coloured pencils or pens place a circle around the words or phrases that you think are the ones being asked for:

1. Circle in red the items that you think are soluble in fat.
2. Circle in green the food items that contain dietary fibre
3. Circle in blue the food items containing amino acids
4. Circle in yellow the water-soluble vitamin components of foods

beta carotene   thiamine   hemicellulose   eggs

menaquinone   whole-wheat bread

lemon juice   riboflavin   α-tocopherol   celery

breakfast Müsli   peanut butter   pantothenate

retinol   tofu   olive oil   magnesium

cholecalciferol   sunflower seeds   yoghurt

ascorbic acid   palmitate   oranges

sardines   phytonutrient

NB: There are five items listed that do not fall into any category

Preventing Disease with Food

Many of the chronic diseases mentioned in the previous learning session are preventable, and the main source of prevention is the improvement of healthy eating and physical activity. These are the two goals of the World Health Organisation (WHO) global strategy on diet, physical activity and health [4]. The cost-effectiveness of prevention of disease by nutritional means cannot be underestimated as both numbers of cardiovascular disorder patients and the cost of treating them with medication and surgery soar [8].

Hypertension is one of the most prevalent problems in Westernised societies, and an emerging epidemic in middle income and developing countries [12], it is the major precursor to a stroke. Diet and lifestyle have a substantial impact on the problem of hypertension with being overweight, physical inactivity, high sodium intake and low potassium intake being the main contributors [12]. The use of diet, however, with no medication could, according to some researchers, reduce the incidence of all types of cardiovascular disease, including that of hypertension and stroke by up to 75%[12,27].

Upon the conclusion of a four-year research project, the American Institute of Cancer Research concluded that the most appropriate approach to the prevention of cancer by dietary means is the consumption of a whole food diet within the context of existing cultural cuisines [10]. This is extremely important in light of the fact that many preventable deaths worldwide are due to the incidence of nutrition induced cancer [28].

In a major study conducted between Cornell University USA and the Chinese Academy of Preventative Medicine, it was found that the same principles of good nutrition, consumption of unprocessed whole foods of vegetable origin and moderate amounts of protein alongside appropriate fat intake were responsible for the prevention of many chronic diseases. The diet that prevented cardiovascular disease was also the same diet that prevented many types of cancer, obesity, type 2 diabetes and osteoporosis [29]. Such dietary principles, alongside a prudent amount of exposure to sunlight in order to obtain an adequate amount of vitamin D, was found to be not only beneficial to health in the short term but also to promote long-term wellbeing and prevent the type of disorders often associated with ageing [29].

Such studies have major implications for the future well-being of the general population. If adherence to general principles of eating can prevent illness across a broader spectrum, it means that an individualised or highly specialised programme of nutrition may not be required by the majority of people [12,13,29]. Although there are variations in what may appear to be recommended, this mainly concerns the amounts of proteins and fats; however, the general principle of obtaining these predominantly from vegetable sources, where possible, is no longer under dispute. This simplifies matters greatly for both the health care professions as well as the ordinary person. Dietary planning need not be complicated, and by adhering to a few well-researched principles, it is possible to use tools and planning guides to construct one's own long-term programme. This will be dealt with in the next learning session.

Learning Together

Activity 2: Allow yourselves 15 minutes for this activity

Do not be daunted if you have not done a crossword before, do this in a group where one of you has done crosswords or ask your facilitator to help you.

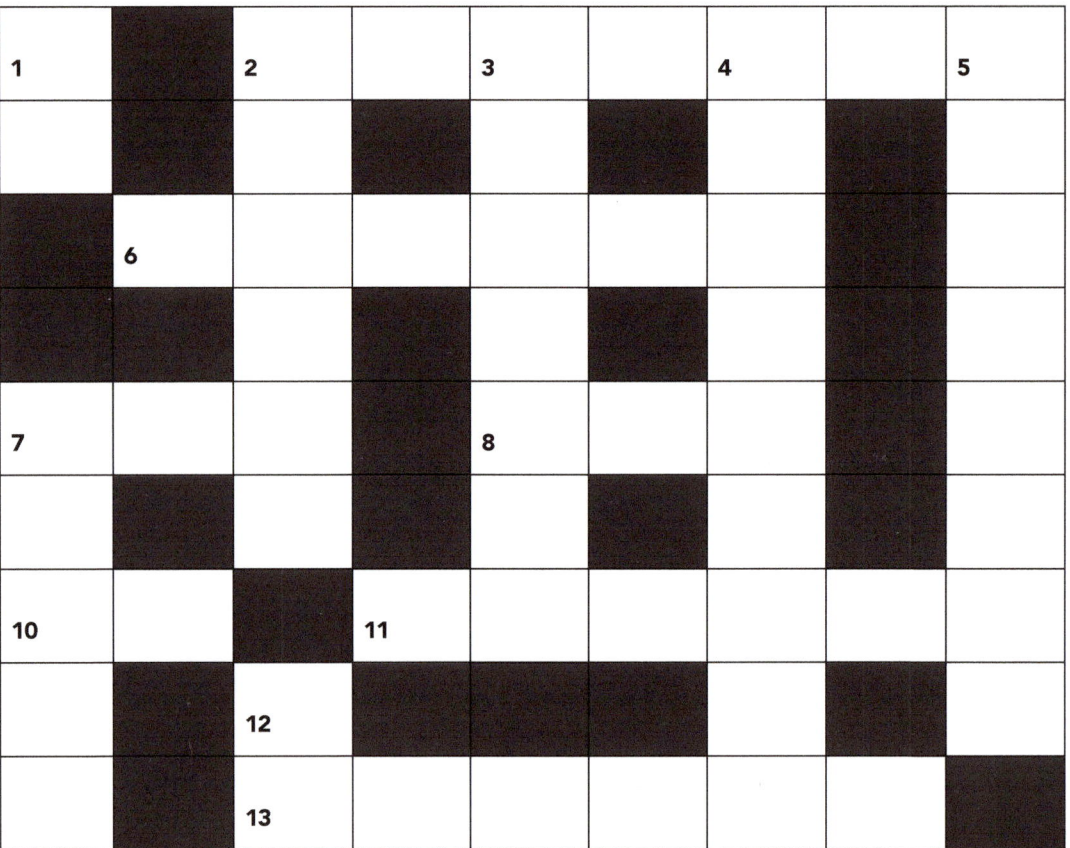

Clues:

Across

2. A macronutrient composed of amino acids
6. If you do not control this problem, the result could be hypertension (high blood pressure) and other illnesses
7. A controversial macronutrient which many feel we could do with less of!
8. The elemental minerals are in this form
10. The chemical abbreviation for the mineral boron
11. An essential amino acid
13. An essential mineral and a constituent of vitamin B12

Down

1. Two fat-soluble vitamins that are not synthesised in the body and need to be taken in with food
2. A well-known vegetable rich in starch
3. A major chronic disorder that has recently risen to epidemic proportions
4. The term used for a nutrient that we cannot do without and which we can only acquire through nutrition
5. The element that is in amino acids but not carbohydrate or fatty acids
7. The substance which is not a nutrient but nevertheless essential to health and found only in vegetable matter
12. The two water soluble vitamins

Now you should take 5 minutes to discuss the answers.

Group Discussion

MALNUTRITION IN MODERN SOCIETIES

Westernised, high income, societies appear to have an abundance of food, and more and more people are suffering from the obesity epidemic. Despite this, many are becoming ill due to lack of vitamins and minerals and obesity is now co-existent alongside nutritional deficiencies. This is also an emerging problem in middle-income countries such as Southern African and South American countries, where overweight exists alongside nutritional deficiency.

Some questions to think about include the following:

- Are people, in general, eating too much overall or just too much of the wrong foods and not enough of the more nutritious items?

- As a group, do you think that this is generally a big problem, or do you think that the problem is overemphasised by the media and the government?

- Alternatively, do you think the problem is bigger than we thought and the focus of attention on it has come a little too late?

- If you think there is a problem in this area, what could you suggest as solutions?

References

1. Murray MT, Pizzorno JE. Nutritional Medicine. In: Pizzorno JE, Murray MT (eds). The Textbook of Natural Medicine. 3rd ed. Volume 1. St Louis: Churchill Livingstone Elsevier, 2006.

2. Merriam-Webster. Merriam-Webster's Medical Dictionary Accessed 2006 26th October. Merriam-Webster Incorporated, 2002.

3. Ashwell M. Concepts of Functional Foods. Brussels: International Life Sciences Institute Europe, 2002.

4. WHO. Diet, Nutrition and the Prevention of Chronic Diseases: Report of a Joint WHO/FAO Expert Consultation. Geneva: World Health Organisation, 2003.

5. WHO. Reducing Risks Promoting Healthy Life. Geneva: World Health Organisation, 2002.

6. Ettinger S. Macronutrients: Carbohydrates, Proteins and Lipids. In: Mahan LK, Escott-Stump S (eds). Krause's Food Nutrition & Diet Therapy. 11th ed. Philadelphia: Saunders Elsevier, 2004.

7. Sackheim GL, Lehman DD. Chemistry for the Health Sciences. 2nd ed. New York: Macmillan; 1994.

8. Olivier S. Eat Your Heart Out. Nursing Standard. 2000;15(9):20-3.

9. Service FJ. Hypoglycaemias. Western Journal of Medicine. 1991;154:442-54.

10. Food, Nutrition and the Prevention of Cancer, a Global Perspective. Washington DC: World Cancer Research Fund / American Institute for Cancer Research, 1997.

11. Brookes L. New Dietary Advice, a New Government Program, A New Drug and a Truly Novel New BP Measurement Device. Medscape Cardiology. Volume 10, 2006:523827.

12. Franco OH, Bonneaux L, de Laet C, Peeters A, Steyerberg EW, Machenbach JP. The Polymeal: a more natural, safer and probably tastier (than the polypill) strategy to reduce cardiovascular disease by more than 75%. British Medical Journal. 2004;329:1447-50.

13. Frassetto L, Morris RC, Sellmeyer DE, Todd K, Sebastian A. Diet, evolution and ageing: The pathophysiological effects of the post-agricultural inversion of potassium-to-sodium and base-to-chloride ratios in the human diet. European Journal of Nutrition. 2001;40(5):200-13.

14. Barclay L, Lie D. High Dietary Antioxidant Intake May Reduce Risk for Age-Related Macular Degeneration. Medscape Medical News. 2006(520823).

15. Campbell MK. Biochemistry. 2nd ed. Orlando: Saunders; 1995.

16. Ettinger S. Macronutrients: Carbohydrates, Proteins and Lipids. In: Mahan LK, Escott-Stump S (eds). Krause's Food, Nutrition & Diet Therapy. 11th ed. Philadelphia: Saunders - Elsevier, 2004.

17. Krummel DA. Medical Nutrition Therapy in Cardiovascular Disease. In: Mahan LK, Escott-Stump S (eds). Krause's Food, Nutrition & Diet Therapy. 11th ed. Philadelphia: Saunders Elsevier, 2004.

18. Crawford MA. The role of dietary fatty acids in biology; their place in the evolution of the human brain. Nutrition Reviews. 1992(50):3.

19. Brooks N, Layne JE, Gordon PL, Roubenoff R, Nelson ME, Castaneda-Sceppa C. Strength training improves muscle quality and insulin sensitivity in Hispanic older adults with type II diabetes. International Journal of Medical Science. 2007;4(1):19-27.

20. WHO. Energy and protein requirements report of a joint FAO/WHO/UNU expert consultation. Geneva: World Health Organisation, 1985.

21. FAO/WHO. Expert consultation on protein quality evaluation. Rome: Food and Agricultural Organisation, 1990.

22. Gallagher ML. Vitamins. In: Mahan LK, Escott-Stump S (eds). Krause's Food Nutrition & Diet Therapy. 11th ed. Philadelphia: Saunders Elsevier, 2004.

23. Anderson JJB. Minerals. In: Mahan LK, Escott-Stump S (eds). Krause's Food, Nutrition & Diet Therapy. 11th ed. Philadelphia: Saunders Elsevier, 2004.

24. Beyer P. Digestion, Absorption, Transport and Excretion of Nutrients. In: Mahan LK, Escott-Stump S (eds). Krause's Nutrition, Diet & Food Therapy. 11th ed. Philadelphia: Saunders Elsevier, 2004.

25. Murray MT, Bongiorno PB. Role of Dietary Fibre in Health and Disease. In: Pizzorno JE, Murray MT (eds). Textbook of Natural Medicine. 3rd ed. Volume 1. St Louis: Churchill Livingstone Elsevier, 2006.

26. Jensen MK, Koh-Bannergee P, Hu FB, et al. Intakes of whole grains, bran, and germ and the risk of coronary heart disease in men. The American Journal of Clinical Nutrition. 2004(80):1492-9.

27. Geleijnse JM, Kok FJ, Grobbee DE. Impact of dietary and lifestyle factors in the prevalence of hypertension in Western populations. European Journal of Public Health. 2004;14(3):235-9.

28. Murray CJL, Lopez AD. The global burden of disease: a comprehensive assessment of mortality and disability from diseases, injuries and risk factors in 1990 and projected to 2020. In: Bank WHOW (ed): Harvard School of Public Health, 1996.

29. Campbell TC, Campbell TM. The China Study: The Most Comprehensive Study of Nutrition Ever Conducted and the Startling Implications for Diet, Weight Loss and Long-term Health: Benbella Books; 2006.

LEARNING SESSION THREE: THE COLOUR WHEEL

Introduction

We discover in this session one of the tools we can use to put our new-found knowledge and understanding together, to create our own guide towards a healthy eating programme. We explore firstly the use of various designs and tools used to plan food intakes, such as the food pyramids and national guidelines. We discuss the advantages and considerations of these and look at how they differ according to their aims and use. We also explore the 'Colour Wheel' and see why and how the focus of this is different. We then move on to explore portions, sizes, and what constitutes an item of food; in other words, what or how much exactly is 'one'?

Our first learning session explores how we know what our own needs are for energy intake and how we work out our personal requirements. Then we move on to the timing of foods, meals and snacks as well as how this affects how our body uses food. In addition, we gain an understanding of why breakfast is so important and how to get over the problem of that feeling of 'just can't face it' early morning lack of appetite.

In the learning session that follows, we are going to create our own plan. After this we move on to our group discussion where we ask the question, do we love ourselves or don't we? The topic of our discussion today is the question of knowing one's own worth. How much are you worth and are you giving yourself all you deserve or are you your own worst enemy?

Ice-Breaker Quiz

This session looks at food balance, appropriate portion sizes and the issue of breakfast, is it really the most important meal of the day or can it be skipped? Let's see how much you might already know – you can do this again later after the session and see the difference in your answers, but for now, look at the list below and, based on the information you have at present:

a. Underline in green the breakfasts you feel might be appropriate for someone with little early morning appetite or not used to eating breakfast

b). Underline in red the meals that you feel are an inappropriate amount   of food or unsuitable for breakfast

c). Underline in yellow the breakfast items that are realistic for someone on a healthy nutrition programme that has a reasonable appetite

d). Underline in blue the breakfasts that are light, but not very nutritious

1. Two fried eggs, bacon, sausage and chips

2. Muesli with plain yoghurt and a piece of chopped fresh fruit

3. Fresh orange juice and a small bowl of stewed apple

4. Two chocolate digestive biscuits and coffee with milk and sugar

5. Blended banana with apple juice and yoghurt

6. Three egg, cheese and onion omelette, fried tomato and French toast

7. A caramel cereal bar and orangeade

8. Two slices of wholegrain toast with unsweetened peanut butter and a piece of fresh fruit

Using Tools in a Nutritional Programme

Creating your own nutritional programme is not as difficult as it sounds, and it will be of added benefit in that it is one that is right for you and takes into consideration your own circumstances, lifestyle, culture and resources. Such resources include those inherent in ourselves and our culture and as discussed in the first session include factors that are pre-disposing, (knowledge gained through both culture and education), enabling, (those that are based in current education and access to health care resources), and reinforcing, (those that help a person keep to a healthy lifestyle, such as support of friends and structured systems of health and well-being) [1].

Certain parts of plants may be more acceptable in some cultures than in others, and every culture will have its own way of preparing these items for eating [2]. Similarly, knowledge passed down the generations of what makes a person feel good or ill, or helps heal certain ailments, will also form part of the cultural cuisine. Sometimes such knowledge is helpful and has been recently scientifically verified. Sometimes this is not helpful and is borne of myth rather than fact [2]. An Australian study found that community support and community-based programmes have been of great value in enhancing health. It has been proposed that community-based action, peer support and social marketing of the benefits of good nutrition may be the way of the future in disease prevention [4,5].

Reinforcing factors: tools we can use

Reinforcing factors are very important in any health and lifestyle management programme. We can have all the knowledge in the world and the best of intentions but, without a structured 'reminder' system and a definite programme to stick to, it is very difficult to manage any ongoing change for a significant length of time. More than 40 nutrients are required in the human diet, and the only sure way of getting all of them in a reasonably utilisable quantity is to have as wide a variety of foods that have been as minimally processed and refined as possible [2]. Advertising has a huge impact on what we buy, and there have never been so many food choices available [5], the problem being that many of these items are made up of similar ingredients thus, even with a large choice available, the ingredients may limit the dietary intake. Social marketing, however, can be a force for good when healthy eating habits are reinforced. Research has found that with awareness and enhanced knowledge, even eating out can be healthy [5].

Numerous standards serve as guides for both evaluating current national food intakes and planning and evaluating diets of both individuals and groups of people. Many countries have issued national guidelines which they believe are appropriate for the circumstances and needs of their respective populations [6]. There are some helpful tools that aid in planning a nutritional programme and reminding us of what our intake should ideally be which have, for many years, been available to dieticians. More recently, some have now been revamped and made available in two forms to the public; these are the various versions of the food pyramid and the food exchange system that we will now discuss [6].

The food pyramid

Various countries, including the UK, US, Canada and Australia, have food guide pyramids. Some give the number of portions per day of the recommended foods, but others do not; they just indicate the ratios of recommended foods. Essentially these translate the national dietary guidelines and nutritional recommendations of the country into a visual form that is user-friendly. The US Food Pyramid is given here (figures are for daily portions):

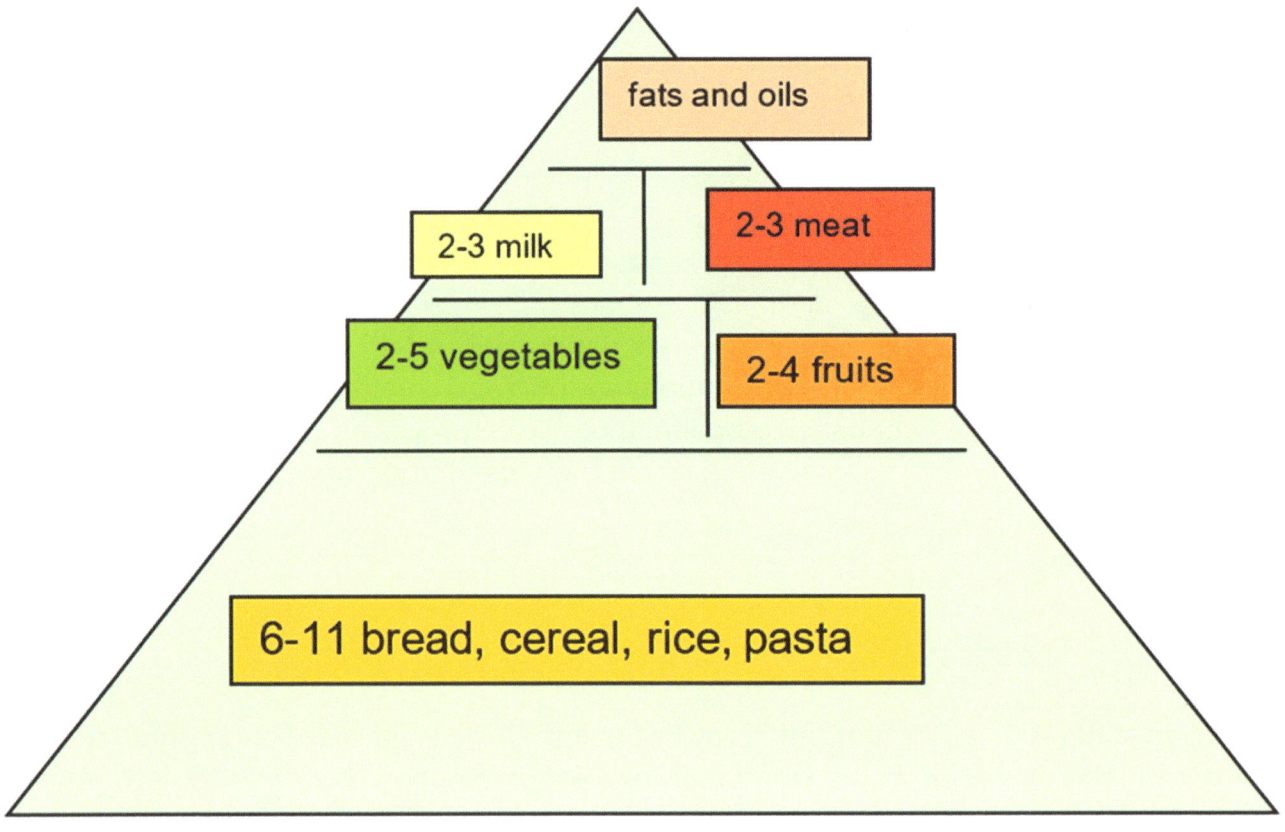

Adapted from: The Food Guide Pyramid US Department of Agriculture and US Department of Health and Human Services [7].

The Children's version of this same pyramid allows for 6 servings of bread and cereals, 3 vegetables, 2 fruits, 2 portions of milk, 2 portions of meat and sparing amounts of fats and sweets [6].

- The main advantages are:
    - Viewing information in a pictorial form tends to make it clearer for the majority of people
    - It is easy to remember
    - This form of information is user-friendly and not overwhelming or off-putting
    - It enhances the concept of balance and proportion between types of foods in the 'ideal' diet

- The main considerations are:
  - There is no international consistency, and there are different versions of the food pyramid in different countries
  - Commercial sponsorship is often involved in the advertising of the food pyramids that influence what type of foods are given as examples
  - There is no distinction between whole foods and processed foods (between white and whole grain bread, for example).
  - In some pyramids (the UK) and the Canadian rainbow concept, there are no guidelines given as to the proportion of fruit to vegetables recommended, and they are viewed as a single food group despite having differing carbohydrate components and differing types of micronutrient content.

The Colour Wheel

This is a tool, which focuses on what you can eat and should be eating and not on what you should not be eating. It focuses on the ratio of macronutrients as well as obtaining the minimum micronutrients. The secret of the colour wheel is that it looks at proportions; therefore, your diet cannot get out of balance. It works by not only looking at the correct ratios of carbohydrate to protein to fat but also at the requirements for fat-soluble and water-soluble nutrients, ratios of $\dot{\omega}3{:}\dot{\omega}6{:}\dot{\omega}9$ and the storage and self-manufacturing capabilities of the body.

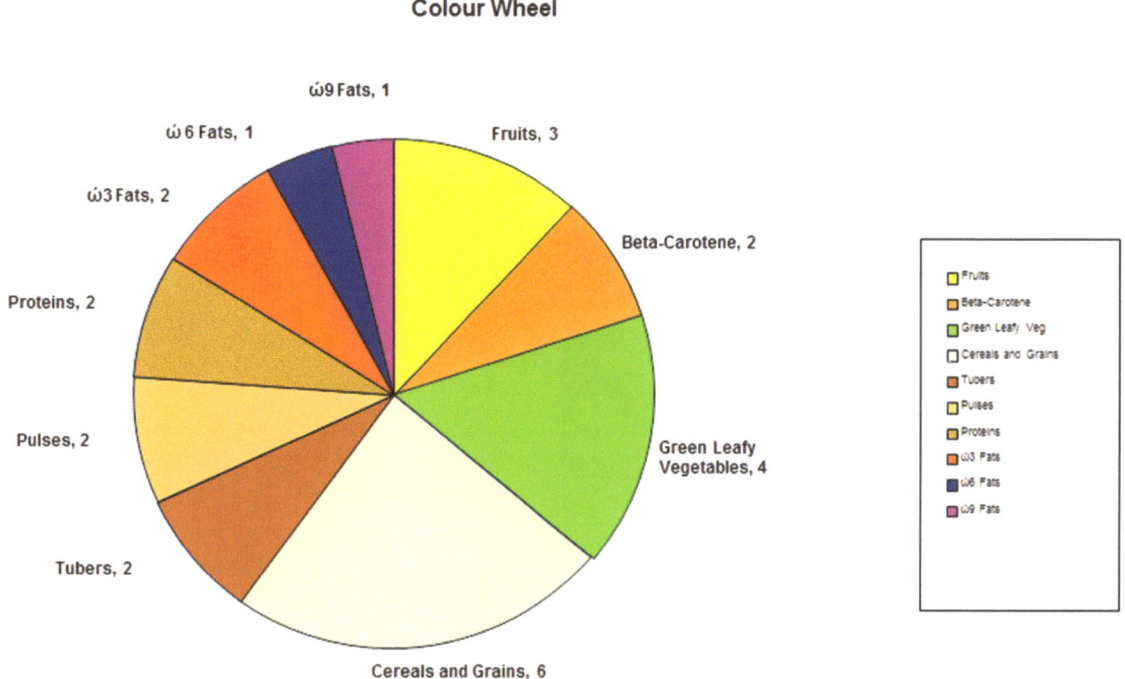

Colour Wheel

Source: author's own construction

NB: This chart gives the ratio of ώ6: ώ3: ώ9 as 1:2:1 for fat portions. As discussed in session 2, it was recommended that one takes in the ratio 1:3:1. One should be aware that there is also considerable ώ6 fatty acid content in the proteins of animal origin such as meats, chicken and dairy products as well as grains and the main source of ώ3 is found in fish for many people.

The colour wheel is much more structured than other food guides and attempts to focus on nutrition as opposed to weight, or calories. This chart is not commercially influenced and is based on the Food and Agricultural Organisation and WHO guidelines for the minimum requirements for energy, protein and nutrients, for adults. The focus is on providing enough micronutrients for the prevention of chronic diseases and the maintenance of health as opposed to losing weight or controlling calories [8]. It aims to meet the recommendations of the WHO / FAO by increasing the intake of fruits and vegetables, increasing the intake of fish and ώ3 fatty acids and changing the types of fats and the ratios of fats consumed. This guide also aims to decrease and discourage the use of other animal proteins, especially red meats, as per WHO recommendations [8].

A controversial issue is that there is no dairy food group listed. This can be taken as part of the protein complement, but it is not a disaster if it is not taken at all as calcium the predominant mineral found in dairy products, can also be found in other foods such as broccoli and sardines. Bone health is vitally important as is the provision for the nutrients that support it. In recent years the spotlight has moved away from the sole provision of large amounts of calcium to support the building of bones as it is now acknowledged that other factors are just as, if not more, important such as ώ-3 fatty acids, vitamin K and vitamin D [9]. Although calcium is important, dairy products may not be the best way of obtaining calcium as absorption depends on other factors such as the presence of magnesium, phosphorous, boron and potassium in the diet, all of which are obtained from grains, nuts and vegetables [10]. Research has shown that an appropriate ώ-3 fatty acid intake is inversely linked with bone resorption which is decreased in the presence of adequate amounts of this nutrient, especially when derived from plant products such as flaxseed (linseed) oil and walnuts [9]. In addition, an adequate amount of D_3 either from sunlight, foods or supplementation is also important in maintaining the growth of bone and reducing its resorption [9]. Protein from plant sources rather than animal sources preserves bone density and lessens its reduction long term.

Portions and Sizes: How Much is 'One'?

Standard serving sizes of foods are set by governments, based usually on reference amounts of foods commonly consumed by the general public [6]. This means that what is consumed in a given population is taken as a reference amount for comparison of nutritional values as opposed to what ought to be consumed. In addition, in different countries, there will be varying ideas of what a commonly consumed amount is and different cultures within a given country may or may not consider that same amount of food 'a portion'.

Nutrition fact labels are slightly more helpful in that they give the nutritional values per portion as well as defining what the manufacturer means by 'a portion,' i.e. ½ can, or 100 g, or 2 crackers, etc. Often the percentage of a nutrient in relation to the daily value or recommended amount is given in addition. As this one nutritional standard may not apply to everyone, however, this may not be a useful measure [6]. How much a portion is depends on who is measuring the portion and what is being measured. Since the government tends to take 'typically eaten' portions as a standard measure, this may well change with circumstances. Research has shown that when we are exposed to education and made aware of the importance of fruit and vegetables, as well as having a little motivation, people ate more fruit and vegetables. Not only was an increased variety consumed but also the quantity was increased [9,11]. A portion, therefore, can be quite literally 'a moveable feast'. Calls have been made for changes in food labelling and for an increased awareness of the quality of foods consumed as opposed to the quantity. In order to meet the 2010 goals for Healthy People, some scientists feel that there should be a greater emphasis on the consumption of fresh foods and unrefined foods, rather than the reliance on portion sizes [12].

The group of international scientists who produced the expert report for the WHO/ FAO have also recommended a change in emphasis globally, from recommendations which are restrictive and calorie / food exchange based, to ones which are based on the quality of intake and are likely to fulfil micronutrient requirements [8]. This means, in effect, that it might be better to define a portion as the practically consumable amount of a given food that would contain a useful quantity of micronutrients. The food pyramids, food rainbow and the food exchange list, do focus on a specific calorific value as well as the macronutrient content for a portion of food but are not always realistic.

The number of portions in the colour wheel is based on a reasonably edible portion of unprocessed micronutrient dense food and taken together will provide between 1,600 and 2,100 Calories per day. Below the 1,600 Calorie mark, it is extremely difficult, if not impossible, to construct a diet which can provide the essential nutrients for a healthy adult without compromising health or necessitating the intake of supplements [13].

The group of international scientists who produced the expert report for the WHO/FAO have also recommended a change in emphasis globally, from recommendations which are restrictive, and calorie or food exchange based, to ones which are based on the quality of food intake and are likely to fulfil all of one's micronutrient requirements [8]. This means, in effect, that it might be better to define a portion as the practically consumable amount of a given food that would contain a useful quantity of micronutrients. This depends on one's own physiology, a good guide being your own right hand, which is proportional to your height and bone structure [14]. The general rule is:

> Curl your right hand – whatever fits into the hollow of the palm = 1 fat
> Whatever you can pick up and hold in a closed hand = 1 grain (uncooked grab and pick up)
> Whatever can fit into the flat palm of your hand 1 little finger thick = 1 protein (not overlapping the base of your fingers)
> Whatever you can hold in your hand with fingers stretched apart = 1 vegetable or fruit

Learning Together

Activity 3.1: Allow yourselves 15 minutes for this exercise

To work out your BMI divide your weight in Kg by your height in Meters squared: E.g., Height = 1.62 m and weight 53 Kg
BMI = 53÷ (1.62 x 1.62) = 53 ÷ 2.62 = 20.229 or 20.23

Write Your BMI down here   _____

BMI Score Result

Less than	18.5	Underweight
	18.5 – 24.9	Correct body mass range
	25.0 – 29.9	Overweight
	30.0 +	Obese

Hip to Waist Ratio Result (Risk of Metabolic Syndrome)

Determine your waist to hip ratio by placing a measuring tape snugly around your waist, and then around the largest part of your hips. This ratio is a good indicator of your abdominal fat, which is a good predictor of your risk for developing risk factors for heart disease and other diseases such as metabolic syndrome and adult-onset diabetes. Measure in inches or centimetres (1 inch = 2.54 cm)

Write your waist measurement down here   _____
Write your hip measurement down here   _____
Divide the hip measurement by the waist measurement   _____

Women	Men	
1.4	1.2	Low risk
1.2	1.1	Moderate risk
1.1 or less	1.0 or less	High risk

Now you should take 5 minutes to discuss the answers

Timing Meals and the Importance of Breakfast

The body's metabolism is like a well-run machine when it has fuel that is. Like any other piece of complex equipment, it cannot run effectively on empty and, given nothing for long enough, it, of course, will not run at all. The metabolism is connected to one's own biorhythms, which in turn are connected to the pattern of light and dark. During darkness, the body naturally slows down the processes of building energy and begins to repair, grow new cells and detoxify the system. As the light slowly begins to affect the system, these processes come to an end, and the business of creating energy for work begins [15].

Originally the eating pattern of humans was to gather food throughout the day, hunting (mainly fish) in the months when nuts, berries and roots were more scarce [16,17]. The metabolism was built for a mainly plant-based diet, high in dietary fibre (with occasional animal products), eaten in small manageable amounts on a frequent basis [16]. There is no evidence to the contrary, and things have not suddenly changed just because of commuting, office hours, or cafeteria opening times.

The ideal time to consume food, it would appear, is during the daylight hours and on a regular ongoing basis. The more frequently one eats, the better the body can burn the food, control the steady flow of glucose into the bloodstream, utilise the nutrients and provide us with sustained energy. In addition, taking in whole, unprocessed foods of vegetable origin with a good measure of fibre / NSP has been shown to prevent excessive circulating glucose concentrations and thus also prevent high amounts of circulating insulin which carry this glucose into the adipose tissue. This, in turn, has been shown not only to decrease fat deposition but data indicate that replacement of 5.4% of total dietary carbohydrate with NSP significantly increased lipid oxidation and therefore could decrease fat accumulation in the long-term [18].

Breakfast is critical to metabolism, and without breakfast, the metabolic rate drops, leading to impaired usage of a normal calorific amount of food. In effect, the less one eats, particularly early in the day, the more the body compensates, lowering the requirement for calories by slowing down the metabolic rate. Unfortunately, this also slows down the rate of repair of tissues and the rate of build-up of immune resources. In addition, depression decreased resistance to stress and cold as well as an increased propensity to illness and higher BMI with increased propensity to obesity has been found in those who either skipped breakfast completely or ate breakfast on an irregular basis [19]. The effect of starting school or work without breakfast is costly and has been shown to affect the results of school tests quite adversely [20]. Research has demonstrated that not eating breakfast results in a lowered ability to take in and process information. More mistakes are made in completing complex tasks, decision making and recall of information [20].

Some people, however, feel that they cannot eat breakfast and are simply not hungry in the morning. This could be due to several factors that have nothing to do with breakfast *per se* but could be because one has eaten late the previous night and has not digested the evening's food. If one has a pattern of going hungry all day and only eating one large meal at night, there is not enough energy to digest that meal and not enough digestive enzymes either. This leads to food leaving the stomach and gastrointestinal system more slowly; thus, it might only be the next morning before this process is complete; hence, one is not hungry. This could turn into a vicious cycle, resulting in low energy levels and obesity. In order to break the pattern, it would be best to choose one day when one does not eat at night, take in plenty of fluids and begin again fresh the next morning with a light breakfast.

Other solutions include:
- Beginning with fresh fruit which metabolises quickly and following this with a high fibre cereal 2-3 hours later
- Beginning with a blender breakfast of fresh fruit and yoghurt which contains a mixture of medium glycaemic and low glycaemic foods as well as bifidoflora which help complete digestion in the lower intestine
- Beginning with water and fresh juice and then going for a pre-breakfast walk to encourage an increase in metabolism and build up an appetite

Many people feel that by skipping meals, they are eating less, or that counting calories and sticking to a strict regimen will result in long term weight loss. Research, however, has shown that this is simply not true. Strict low-calorie regimens are difficult to maintain and often unhealthy. The US Dept of Agricultural Science evaluated some popular weight loss diets and, in fact, found that regardless of the type of diet, all of them resulted in short term weight loss. Some of the weight loss, especially on the low carbohydrate diets was water rather than fat, no diet was optimal in reducing hunger, and some diets over the long term resulted in nutritional deficiencies [21]. Given that it is virtually impossible to plan a well-balanced diet that will prevent disease which is less than 1,600 Cal per day, and that even a 5% to 10% weight loss will result in many health benefits, calorie counting *per se* may not, in fact, be necessary [21].

Advocates of the non-diet approach to food intake, focus on setting health goals as opposed to weight goals. This programme focusses on eating for disease prevention and energy maintenance as opposed to 'dieting'. This non-diet paradigm maintains that the body will achieve its own natural weight if the individual eats healthily, becomes attuned to satiety and hunger cues and incorporates physical activity into their lives [21]. The process of attuning to satiety and hunger is paramount for this approach to work at all, which brings us back to the question of frequency of eating and the golden rule is eat something when you are hungry and nothing when you are not.

Quick Quiz

Do you recognise the food groups in the 'colour wheel'? On the left is a list of foods and on the right is a list of food groups – draw a line linking each food to one of the food groups. Use coloured pencils for each food group link.

Cabbage

Carrots   ώ 3 rich fats

Olives

Lentils   ώ 6 rich fats

Bananas

Pilchards   ώ 9 rich fats

Sweet potatoes

Cauliflower   Green Vegetables

Sunflower seeds

Porridge oats   Beta Carotene Foods

Apricots

Broccoli   Fruit

Almonds

String Beans   Grains

Couscous

Kidney Beans   Tubers

Apples

Salmon   Pulses

Brown rice   Proteins

English Walnuts

Plums

Linseeds (Flaxseeds)

Whole Maize (Corn on the Cob)

Canola oil

Watercress

Finding the Right Balance for You

Whether or not you use the food pyramid, national guidelines or the 'colour wheel', you need to take your own personal needs into consideration. This means that you need to look at where and how you personally might be vulnerable to disease and whether certain disease traits appear to run in your family.

As this is a health maintenance and health enhancement programme as opposed to a weight loss plan we are opting to guide you through the non-diet, disease prevention approach to customising the 'colour wheel' for yourself. This does not prevent you from taking advantage of other tools or other approaches if you feel that they are more appropriate to your immediate requirements. In essence, the basis of a healthy balanced nutritional programme which is plant-based and unprocessed will solve most common health problems where nutritional imbalances are directly the cause, or a major contributing factor, as well as preventing many nutrition-related disorders [22].

Persons who are hypertensive, or at risk for hypertension and stroke should be mindful to lower the sodium content and increase the potassium content of their diet by not limiting the amount of fresh vegetables consumed [23-26]. Persons who are obese, at high risk for metabolic syndrome and have a family history of cardiovascular disease or arthritic conditions should reduce the ώ6 fat content of the diet and increase the ώ3 fat content of the diet by exchanging meat for cold water fish [25,27]. Persons at risk for either cardiovascular disease or adult-onset type 2 diabetes would benefit from increasing the fibre content of the diet by ensuring that grains are consumed as whole food products and not refined and processed products [27,28,29]. Anyone with a blood glucose problem, be it diabetes or hypoglycaemia, needs to be especially aware of the timing of foods and to plan not only what they eat but when they eat, incorporating not only the principles of good nutrition into their programme but also those of regular eating patterns and healthy snacks [30,31].

This necessity of increasing the fibre content of the diet equally holds true for those at risk or with a family history of colorectal cancer, as does the necessity for increasing vegetables, especially those rich in beta carotene [32-34]. Those at risk for infection or who have altered immune deficiency states as well as persons who have had frequent use of antibiotics or are at increased risk of cardiomyopathy, should they contract a bacterial infection (such as those with a mitral valve prolapse) would be best including plenty of antioxidant containing foods such as fruits, vegetables, avocado pears and brazil nuts. This holds true for those who smoke as well, as the antioxidants, especially vitamin C, are utilised in far greater quantities by those who smoke [22,32].

Women at risk for osteoporosis as well as small boned desk bound fair skinned men might benefit from increasing their sources of vitamin D found in cold water fish, and eggs rather than eating meat [35]. Fatty cold-water fish is also beneficial in redressing the acid-alkali balance as is decreasing acid-forming foods that increase the leaching of calcium from bones, such as meat, salt and pickles [9].

The important thing about this programme is that it is, at the end of the day, your own, you need to look to your nutritional requirements first and meet these before you give calories or weight any consideration. Probably, however, a healthy eating plan based on whole foods mainly of vegetable origin, which does not miss out on any major food group is not going to make you increase your weight or body fat. Let us now look at the practical issue of putting at all together in the learning session.

Learning Together

Activity 3.2: Allow yourselves 15 minutes for this activity

This exercise has two parts to it: firstly, take one day's typical food intake and make a comparison with the colour wheel – see how your current intake fits in with what you should be eating. Make a note of where you may be taking in too little and where you may be taking in too much of each of the food categories.

Secondly, you should know your BMI from the previous learning session. Bear in mind that you cannot provide a full nutritionally adequate diet over the long term under 1600 Calories per day, which is the baseline of the 'colour wheel'. If your BMI is between 18.5 and 25, you are not under or overweight, begin your planning at this level on the following page. If you are underweight, you need to ensure that you are eating correctly and have all the required nutrients. If your BMI is over 25, you need to ensure that your intake is balanced and to factor in more exercise rather than less food.

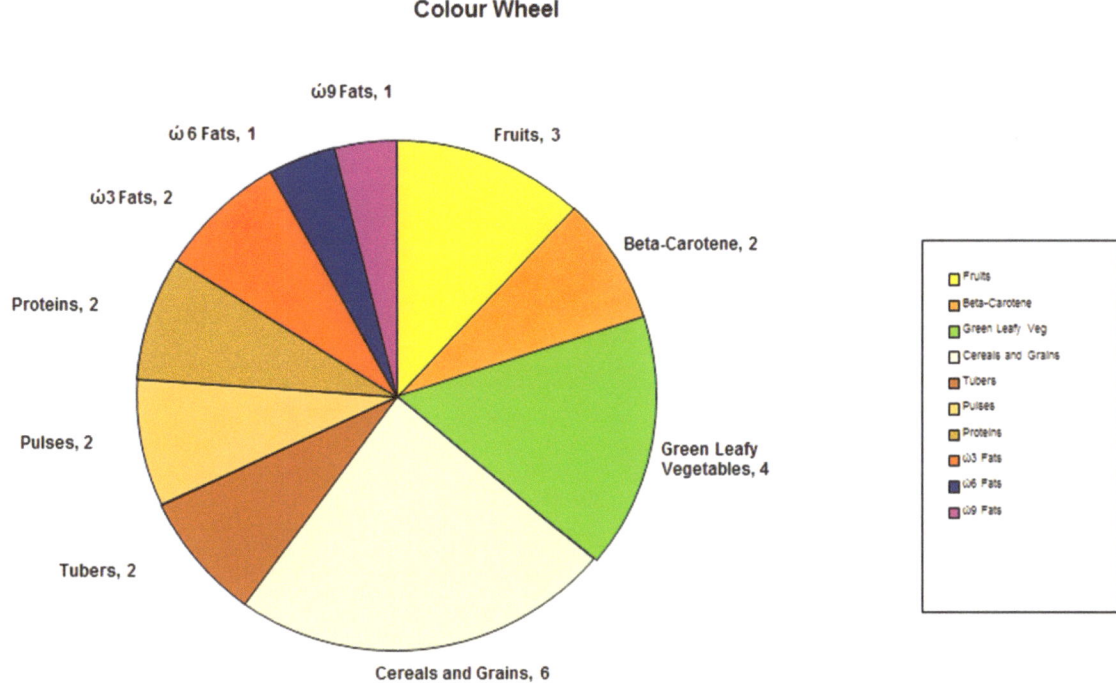

Colour Wheel

Now you can take the reminder sheet and fill in what you should be eating, adding or deducting from your current food intake as per your personal needs.

	Cereals and Grains (brown rice; whole grain pasta; low GI muesli; polenta/ whole grain maize; millet)	Green Leafy Veg (all greens leaves and cabbages; aubergines; marrows; green beans; tomatoes; salad veg)	Beta Carotene (carrots; pumpkin; butternut;)	Fruits (apples; pears; quince; apricots strawberries)	Tubers (potatoes; sweet potatoes; yams; artichokes)	Pulses (beans; lentils; soy products)	Proteins (Fish; skinned poultry; eggs and fermented dairy)	Omega 6 Fats (nuts; avocado pear; seeds; peanut butter)	Omega 9 Fats (olives x3; olive oil; coconut)	Omega 3 fats (walnuts x 3; linseeds; canola oil; walnut oil or extra portion fish = 2 omega 3 fats)
Monday										
Tuesday										
Wednesday										
Thursday										
Friday										
Saturday										
Sunday										
Total for week										
My Total										
Difference										

Group Discussion

DO YOU KNOW YOUR OWN WORTH AND ARE YOU GIVING YOURSELF ALL YOU DESERVE?

This discussion is about value; how much do we really value ourselves and do we reward ourselves with help or harm? Many people have never been taught to value themselves, worse still they reward themselves with damaging things, which in the extreme version could lead to excessive alcohol intake or recreational drug usage. Often, it is damaging foods, those that do nothing for us and might have some taste appeal but detract from our long-term health and happiness. Some questions to think about and discuss group:

- When we reward ourselves for hard work or achievement, how often do we do this with food or drink items as opposed to non-food or drink items?
- If you 'treat' yourself with a large hot chocolate and a piece of rich 'gateau', knowing that there is no long-term benefit, is it really a treat?
- Could this situation fall into a mild 'self-harm' or form of self-sabotage?
- Can we think of items that might be food and drink but are more rewarding nutritionally than damaging?
- Could we feel just as good with a non-food reward such as toiletries, a CD, paperback or a movie ticket?
- Could we find a way of celebrating that is not food or drink focussed?

References

1. Johnson PH, Kittleson MJ. A Qualitative Exploration of Health Behaviours and the Associated Factor among University Students from Different Cultures. The International Electronic Journal of Health Education. Volume 6, 2003:14-25.
2. Truswell AS. ABC of Nutrition: Some Principles. British Medical Journal. 1985;291:1486-90.
3. Black SA. Diabetes, Diversity and Disparity. American Journal of Public Health. 2002;92(4):543-8.
4. Dunt D, Day N, Pirkis J. Evaluation of a community-based health promotion programme supporting public health policy initiatives for a healthy diet. Health Promotion International. 1999;14(4):317-27.
5. Ancharya RN, Patterson PM, Hill EP, Schmitz TG, Bohm E. An Evaluation of the "TrEAT Yourself Well" Restaurant Nutrition Campaign. Health Education and Behaviour. 2006(June):309-24.
6. Earl R. Guidelines for Dietary Planning. In: Mahan LK, Escott-Stump S (eds). Krause's Food Nutrition & Diet Therapy. 11th ed. Philadelphia: Saunders, 2004.
7. Earl R. The Food Guide Pyramid. US Department of Agriculture and US Department of Health and Human Services, 2004:The Food Guide Pyramid.
8. WHO. Diet, Nutrition and the Prevention of Chronic Diseases: Report of a Joint WHO/ FAO Expert Consultation. Geneva: World Health Organisation, 2003.
9. Griel AE, Kris-Etherton PM, Hilpert KF, Zhao G, West SG, Corwin RL. An increase in dietary n-3 fatty acids decreases a marker of bone resorption in humans. Nutrition Journal. Volume 6, 2007.
10. Anderson JJB. Minerals. In: Mahan LK, Stump SE (eds). Krause's Food Nutrition & Diet Therapy. 11th ed. Philadelphia: Saunders Elsevier, 2004.
11. Steptoe A, Perkins-Porras L, McKay C, Rink E, Hilton S, Cappuccio FP. Behavioural counselling to increase consumption of fruit and vegetables in low-income adults: randomised trial. British Medical Journal. 2003;326:855-8.
12. Nestle M, Jacobson MF. Halting the Obesity Epidemic: A Public Health Policy Approach. Public Health Reports. 2000;2000(115):12-24.
13. WHO. Energy and protein requirements report of a joint FAO/WHO/UNU expert consultation. Geneva: World Health Organisation, 1985.
14. Tortora GJ, Derrickson B. Principles of Anatomy and Physiology. 12 ed. Hoboken New Jersey USA: John Wiley & Sons; 2009.
15. Beyer PL. Digestion, Absorption, Transport and Excretion of Nutrients. In: Mahan LK, Escott-Stump S (eds). Krause's Food, Nutrition & Diet Therapy. 11th ed. Philadelphia: Saunders Elsevier, 2004.
16. Frassetto L, Morris RC, Sellmeyer DE, Todd K, Sebastian A. Diet, evolution and ageing: The pathophysiological effects of the post-agricultural inversion of potassium-to-sodium and base-to-chloride ratios in the human diet. European Journal of Nutrition. 2001;40(5):200-13.
17. Oppenheimer S. Out of Eden : The peopling of the world. London: Constable and Robinson; 2004.

18. Higgins JA, Higbee DR, Donahoo WT, Brown IL, Bell ML, Bessensen DH. Resistant starch consumption promotes lipid oxidation. Nutrition and Metabolism. Volume 1, 2004.

19. Yang R-J, Wang EK, Hsieh Y-S, Chen M-Y. Irregular breakfast eating and health status among adolescents in Taiwan. Biomed Central Public Health. Volume 6, 2006.

20. Pollitt E, Mathews R. Breakfast and cognition: an integrative summary. American Journal of Clinical Nutrition. 1998;67(S):804.

21. Laquatra I. Nutrition for Weight Management. In: Mahan LK, Escott-Stump S (eds). Krause's Food Nutrition and Diet Therapy. 11th ed. Philadelphia: Saunders Elsevier, 2004.

22. Campbell TC, Campbell TM. The China Study: The Most Comprehensive Study of Nutrition Ever Conducted and the Startling Implications for Diet, Weight Loss and Long-term Health: Benbella Books; 2006.

23. Brookes L. New Dietary Advice, a New Government Program, A New Drug and a Truly Novel New BP Measurement Device. Medscape Cardiology. Volume 10, 2006:523827.

24. Cook NR, Cutler JA, Obarszanek E, et al. Long term effects of dietary sodium reduction on cardiovascular disease outcomes: observational follow-up of the trials of hypertension prevention (TOHP). British Medical Journal. Volume 334, 2007.

25. Reddy KS, Katan MB. Diet, nutrition and the prevention of hypertension and cardiovascular diseases. Public Health Nutrition. 2004;71(A)(Supplement 1):167-86.

26. Vollmer WM, Sacks FM, Svetkey LP. New insights into the effects on blood pressure of diets low in salt and high in fruits and vegetables and low-fat dairy products. Current Controlled Trials in Cardiovascular Medicine. 2001;2:71-4.

27. Franco OH, Bonneaux L, de Laet C, Peeters A, Steyerberg EW, Machenbach JP. The Polymeal: a more natural, safer and probably tastier (than the polypill) strategy to reduce cardiovascular disease by more than 75%. British Medical Journal. 2004;329:1447-50.

28. Gardner CD, Coulston A, Chatterjee L, Rigby A, Spiller G, Farquhar JW. The Effect of a Plant-Based Diet on Plasma Lipids in Hypercholesterolemic Adults. Annals of Internal Medicine. 2005;145:725-33.

29. Joffe M, Robertson A. The potential contribution of increased vegetable and fruit consumption to health gain in the European Union. Public Health Nutrition. 2001;4(4):893-901.

30. Yannakoulia M. Eating Behavior among Type 2 Diabetic Patients: A Poorly Recognized Aspect in a Poorly Controlled Disease. The Review of Diabetic Studies. Volume 3, 2006.

31. Service FJ. Hypoglycaemias. Western Journal of Medicine. 1991;154:442-54.

32. Cannon G (ed). Food, Nutrition and the Prevention of Cancer: a global perspective. Washington DC: World Cancer Research Fund / American Institute for Cancer Research; 1997.

33. van-Breda SGJ, van-Agen E, Engels LGJB, Moonen EJC, Kleinjans JCS, van-Delft JHM. Altered vegetable intakes affects pivotal carcinogenesis pathways in colon mucosa from adenoma patients and controls. Carcinogenesis 2004;25(11):2207-16.

34. Grimble RF. Nutritional modulation of immune function. Proceedings of the Nutrition Society. 2001;60:389-97.

35. Gallagher JC, Jerpbak CM, Jee WSS, Johnson KA, DeLuca HF, Riggs BL. 1,25-Dihydroxyvitamin D_3 : Short and Long-term effects on bone and calcium metabolism with postmenopausal osteoporosis. Procedures of the National Academy of Sciences USA. 1982;79:3325-9.

LEARNING SESSION FOUR: CIGARETTES AND ALCOHOL, THE VISIBLE AND HIDDEN COSTS

Introduction

Nicotine has in the context of the history of mankind, not been with us for very long but its impact on society, however, has been drastic. Over time nicotine has moved from cultural use to that of haute couture and eventually to social unacceptability. Despite the diminishing popularity of smoking in the developed world, its use is increasing in the developing world. This session looks at the impact of nicotine, physically, psychologically and socially. We review not only the individual health risks but also the economic and environmental impact. In our first learning together session, we ask you to make an informed evaluation of the impact of nicotine yourselves, before moving on to the question of alcohol consumption.

Alcohol is chemically an anaesthetic, but it impacts differently on individuals who use it. We look at the official definition of alcoholism and question the dividing line between heavy drinking and problem drinking. What in fact, is 'responsible drinking'? How much is enough and how much is too much? We review the obvious and hidden costs of drinking and look at some statistics that are not always considered in a full evaluation of the impact of alcohol on society.

Once again in the second learning together session we ask you as a group to make an informed evaluation of the total impact of alcohol on your life, which may be surprising, even if you do not consume it yourself. In the light of medical evidence both for and against the health impact of alcohol consumption, in the final discussion, we question whether there are any benefits, despite the considerations, that we could not obtain from another source?

Ice-Breaker Quiz

1. The global production of Barley is approximately 140 million tonnes, the percentage used for making alcohol is:

Answer: _____

A. less than 0.5%
B. 2%
C. 8%
D. 10% +

2. The global production of all types of grapes exceeds 62 million tonnes, the largest commercial use is for:

Answer: _____

A. cough mixture
B. raisins
C. wine production
D. production of glucose

3. One packet of 20 cigarettes uses up the same amount of vitamin C in the body as is contained in:

Answer: _____

A. 20 cherries
B. 7 large oranges
C. 200 ml orange juice
D. 2 Bloody Mary cocktails

4. Nicotine contains approximately 250 toxic chemicals, the number of these that are carcinogenic (cancer causing) is:

Answer: _____

A. 5
B. 15
C. 25
D. 50

5. The largest alcohol related cause of death is:

Answer: _____

A. Kidney failure
B. Road traffic accidents
C. Alcohol poisoning
D. Wernicke's syndrome

Nicotine: What It Is and What It Does.

The cultivation of tobacco leaf, which was indigenous to the Americas, dates back at least eight hundred years, originally used by Native Americans, Columbus was the first known 'importer' of tobacco into Europe [1] . Found in tobacco leaves, nicotine is chemically a water-soluble alkaloid, and an effective insecticide [2]. Raw tobacco leaves from farmers are dried and cured before they are sold on to a manufacturer for processing into a consumer product [1]. To maximize profits, tobacco manufacturers want to make products that are as attractive as possible [1]. Tobacco has no known therapeutic use but is found in the body after smoking or chewing tobacco. There are over 250 chemical components in cigarette smoke; the most active ingredient is nicotine, which has both pharmacologic and behavioural effects and is highly addictive [3].

In addition to nicotine, smokers may be getting more than they bargained for with significant doses of other chemicals that they may not have been aware of. Cigarettes are highly technical products, and manufacturers are becoming as creative as those of other recreational designer drugs. Today's cigarettes may include leaf stems and tobacco dust and are 'cut' with hundreds of other chemicals diluting down the nicotine content and stretching the profit per dollar [1, 4]. Additives include ammonia and ammonium hydroxide which enhance smoke inhalation, increase absorption of nicotine, and in their own right, damage the respiratory tract [1, 4]. Flavourings, sweeteners as well as cognac oil and rum extract are also added, and it is usually these products as opposed to the type or quality of tobacco used that impart the distinctive brand flavour [1, 4]. Increasingly low quality reconstituted tobacco is used, making the addition of other chemicals easier and the profit margin even greater [1, 4].

Initially, nicotine relaxes the central nervous system, calming the user and decreasing the perception of pain as well as acting as a temporary appetite suppressant [5]. Within minutes, however, despite the behavioural effect, nicotine raises the metabolic rate, thus raising the blood pressure and pulse rate, adding stress to the cardiovascular system and constricting the airways [2]. Simply put, the body works overtime while running on empty, while the brain stops caring about the overload and becomes immune to the working conditions. Nicotine constricts the blood vessels, increasing blood pressure, and pulse rate [2], leading to stroke and heart attacks [6].

The addictive factor in smoking is alarming, out of every 100 people who try cocaine, 18 will become addicts, whereas out of every 100 people who try cigarettes, 90 will become addicts [7]. Commercial cigarettes are a form of designer drug that currently kills 50% of its users [8]. Moreover it is hard to stop, only 15% of smokers who try to give up without assistance remain abstinent after one year; however, nicotine replacement therapy (NRT) counselling and cognitive behaviour treatments are effective [7].

Globally tobacco use is the leading preventable cause of death and disease [1]. Smoking kills more than six million people each year with most deaths occurring from, ischemic heart disease, chronic obstructive pulmonary disease (COPD), lung cancer and chronic airway obstruction [1]. If the current trend continues by 2030, tobacco use will be directly responsible for 8 million deaths annually, mostly in lower and middle-income countries [6]. Aside from heart disease, smoking-related COPD is on the rise. COPD results in declined airflow both in and out of the lungs, but symptoms only begin when the lung capacity has declined in excess of 25% [9]. The prognosis for smokers with COPD is not good, with first symptoms occurring at age 50 the person who continues to smoke will most likely progressively decline in health and die before age 65. Even if one stops smoking at diagnosis, however, up to five years of extra life can be gained [9]. The effects of smoking on pregnancy are almost as alarming as those of alcohol, with a far greater risk of both low birth-weight and low-placental-weight which inhibits the growth development and long-term health of the unborn child [10]. Smoking not only has physiological effects but has recently been linked to schizophrenia and psychosis [11]. Yet, approximately 942 million men and 175 million women globally, continue to smoke cigarettes [1].

Aside from smokers, even non-smokers suffer from the effects of side-stream smoke inhaling up to 25%, i.e. inadvertently smoking one in four of the cigarettes smoked by someone in the same room, vehicle or other immediate air space. An estimated 20% of Men and 33% of women are inadvertently exposed to second-hand smoke from cigarettes, cigars and water-pipes [1]. Recent and comprehensive reviews of the scientific evidence estimated that chronic exposure to second-hand smoke caused approximately 884 000 deaths in 2016 [1]. The collective global years of life lost due to ill-health, disability, or early death because of second-hand smoke was an estimated 6.4 million years in 2016 mainly due to lower respiratory infections, with 2.5 million years lost for chronic obstructive pulmonary disease, and more than 200,000 years lost for middle ear infections [1]. Estimates for heavily populated areas where there is little or no control over smoking in public places could reveal even higher figures for this type of exposure. It appears that there is no safe level of exposure to environmental tobacco smoke. While cigar and pipe smoking have been thought of as safer options, these too, carry risks and have both been linked to pancreatic cancer [12]. Snus, a form of smokeless tobacco does have the benefit of reducing the effects of second-hand smoke for others in the same environment, and moderate reduction of other smoking-related disorders has been found [13]. There are nonetheless concerns that aggressive marketing of snus might encourage its use among those who would not normally smoke [13].

In developing countries, there is an added and direct nutritional burden to the problem of smoking, that of low Body Mass Index (BMI). The BMI of any given person or population is generally a good indicator of nutritional status and overall health [14]. In India, smokers are three times more likely to have a low BMI than non-smokers [5] and tobacco use appears to be an independent indicator of low BMI and poor nutritional status [5] The difference between the BMI of smokers and non-smokers was more pronounced in women than men, which is of concern, especially in women of childbearing age [5]. Reasons for this difference could be two-fold, firstly nicotine affects appetite directly lessening the desire for food; secondly, it lessens the purchasing power of the smoker, thus reducing the household supply of food [5].

Exchanging one type of use for another will do nothing to increase the economic status of tobacco users or their food purchasing power in poorer communities. Despite the spectacular advances being made in the detection and treatment of tobacco-related illness, deaths from tobacco use are currently on the increase and are predicted to rise [1].

Quick Quiz

1. Smoking contributes to approximately how many deaths per year globally?

   Answer: _____

   A. 2 million
   B. 6 million
   C. 8 million
   D. 10 million

2. By 2030 annual deaths due to smoking will have increased / decreased to.

   Answer: _____

   A. 8 million
   B. 5 million
   C. 2 million
   D. 1 Million

3. Apart from nicotine, the following additives are also found in cigarettes:

   Answer: _____

   A. Aluminium hydroxide and cognac
   B. Ammonium and tar
   C. Saccharine and alcohol
   D. Ammonium and Flavourings

4. The percentage of people who try cigarettes that will become addicted to them is:

   Answer: _____

   A. 18%
   B. 20%
   C. 50%
   D. 90%

5. The percentage of people who will die as a result of tobacco use is:

   Answer: _____

   A. 18%
   B. 20%
   C. 50%
   D. 90%

Tobacco, The Environment and The Economy

Tobacco is grown in over 160 countries on more than 4 million hectares of the world's arable land, with only 42 countries confirmed as growing no tobacco growing at all [1]. Currently, the US, Brazil, China and India are the largest producers of tobacco leaf, but lower-income countries such as Indonesia, Kenya Malawi, Philippines, Zambia and Zimbabwe also collectively produce large amounts of tobacco leaf, albeit at a very low-profit margin [1]. Successfully growing tobacco relies heavily on fertiliser and pesticide use and the runoff from this as well as the incessant use of the land for a single crop causes extensive environmental damage [1,4]. On top of this, the curing of tobacco releases chemicals into the atmosphere, damaging fauna and local populations [1,4]. Tobacco agriculture too has effects on those who work in this industry, green tobacco sickness and pesticide poisoning, as well as respiratory damage from tobacco dust, are occupational hazards for many employees [1,4].

In lower-income countries tobacco leaf is grown on contract to large suppliers or commodity agents who dictate both quality and price, leaving the individual farmers with little manoeuvring space to determine how much they receive for their efforts [1]. The success of large-scale tobacco companies is often due to purchasing power and low costs involved in buying cheaply from small-scale farmers in low-income countries [1]. Tobacco production often exists alongside insufficient food production and basic food shortages.

Annually over 5 trillion cigarettes are manufactured with China leading the market followed closely by the USA and India. The China National Tobacco Corporation makes more than one-third of the world's cigarettes, 97% of which is for local consumption. The other two-thirds of the world's cigarettes are made predominantly by six large multinational organisations, the two principal ones being Altria/Phillip Morris and British American Tobacco (BAT). Although the multinationals dabble increasingly in the pharmaceutical, food and drink industry as well, the economic value from nicotine alone amounts to hundreds of billions of dollars with as little as 1% of this going directly to the farmers [1,4]. In recent years the industry has taken advantage of developing countries with cheap labour and few controls, employing approximately 7.5 million persons. Of great concern, however, is the issue of child workers in the tobacco industry. In 2004 Manufacturers in India employed approximately six million children aged between four and fourteen in the tobacco industry mainly hand-rolling bidis (local cigarettes) [4]. Although bidi manufacture has been automated and there has been a major effort to get children into school [1] as of 2018, child labour is still a major problem with approximately 1.2 million children under 15 years of age employed in various sectors of tobacco and cigarette production [15].

Local and international constraints on tobacco growing and manufacturing would be ineffective without the global control of measures that aim to reduce the overall demand [1]. This is a difficult task, and as with any other designer drug, the illegal trade and undercover blocking are both as pervasive as they are profitable. Governments can control consumption and raise considerable amounts of money from tax revenues; however, this is undermined when cigarettes are illicitly smuggled into a country [1]. Cigarettes appear to be the world's most widely smuggled legal consumer product, bypassing both legal restrictions and health regulations [1]. Despite claims to the contrary, it appears that one major transnational organisation has encouraged this illegal tobacco trade through its international agents, in order to deliberately expand its international market, most notably but not exclusively in China, where this market is supposedly under strict governmental control [1]. The main targets of these contraband products are low-income consumers and youth in developing countries, making recognised brands more available and, therefore, more popular [1].

Out of 192 WHO member states and the EU, 167 have signed the WHO Framework Convention on Tobacco Control (FCTC) which came into effect in 2005 [4]. This convention, not surprisingly, ran into disagreement with the tobacco industry which sought voluntary controls and self-regulating market mechanisms [4] The FCTC deals with the reduction in use of tobacco, despite this, however, use of tobacco is destined to rise due to the increase in global population [1], unless more drastic measures of control are sought and implemented. As of 2005 complete bans on smoking were rare but the process of smoking bans were being implemented in private workplace areas [4]. The main beneficiary of workplace smoking bans are employers, as smoking bans are inexpensive to implement, reduce fires, lower insurance premiums and reduce employee absenteeism [1,4].

Learning Together

Activity 4.1: Allow 15 minutes for this exercise

In small working groups, take one of the following issues with the tobacco industry:

a). The use of labour in the industry, who is employed and the amount they are paid;

b). The issue of damage to the environment from the growing of tobacco as well as smoking;

c). The health damage to the individual who uses tobacco or

d). The overall effect of the tobacco industry on the non-smoker.

1. Write down the three largest or most urgent problems connected with one of the above issues in order of importance.

2. Try between you as a group to come up with a possible solution to the most urgent, or largest problem on your list.

Now you should take 5 minutes to discuss the answers

Alcohol, The Ultimate Anaesthetic

The consumption of alcohol among young adults appears to have increased, especially in the UK, USA and some other westernised and rapidly developing regions of the world such as Scandinavia, Eastern Europe and the Western Pacific [16]. The consumption of alcoholic beverages can be studied from several viewpoints, ranging from that of an economist to a social researcher. When viewed from a health perspective, alcoholic beverages can potentially be an agent of illness and mortality. Depending on the consumption pattern, use of alcoholic beverages can elevate the drinker's risk of health problems (traffic and other accidents, chronic illness such as cirrhosis and cancer, and mental disorders such as alcohol dependence) as well as social problems (inability to cope with work, family and other roles, and harm to those in the drinker's surrounding environment) [16].

Ethyl alcohol, (ethanol) is commonly referred to either as potable alcohol or grain alcohol, and it is the most common form of alcohol consumed. It is prepared from the fermentation of blackstrap molasses or the malting of grains. One important activity of this compound is its irreversible ability to denature protein. Because of this, it is widely used as an antiseptic [2]. The concentration of alcohol in beverages is expressed as 'proof' which is twice the percentage of alcohol in the solution; thus, a beverage marked 100% proof contains 50% alcohol [2]. Despite the common and subjective perceptions of the action of alcohol, it is not a stimulant, but a mild anaesthetic and depressant, lowering the speed at which nerve transmission takes place in the central nervous system [2]. Alcohol lowers the body temperature, physical actions slow down, one becomes less coordinated, and normal inhibitions may be removed [2]. Alcohol is also a diuretic, increasing the flow of urine, and if replacing other fluids, may cause moderate to severe dehydration [2].

Acetaldehyde formed from alcohol in the body is responsible for many of the unpleasant side effects of alcohol consumption. The drug Antabuse is used to treat alcohol dependency and functions by increasing the formation of acetaldehyde, thus increasing the unpleasantness of alcohol consumption.

Alcohol use is related to a wide range of physical, mental and social harms. Most health professionals agree that alcohol affects practically every organ in the human body. Alcohol consumption was linked to more than 60 disease conditions in recent studies [16]. The overall consequences depend not only on the quantity of consumption but also on the pattern of consumption and circumstances such as the ability to metabolise alcohol, intoxication and dependency. Approximately 10% of drinkers become dependent on alcohol [7].

The alcohol content of beverages is a key risk factor for its various adverse consequences. The biochemical effects of alcohol are an important factor; in addition to the neurological effects that create conditions for accidents and chemical dependency, there is also the possibility of developing chronic health problems, [16]. With the excessive intake of alcohol, magnesium ions are lost via the urine. Magnesium is an important mineral in the body which is required for more than 100 metabolic reactions [2]. The clinical signs of a magnesium deficiency include tremors, convulsions, delusions, disorientation and extreme irritability often seen in persons who regularly consume large amounts of alcohol [2]. Excessive use of alcohol causes cirrhosis of the liver [2] brought about by hyperlipidaemia and subsequent destruction of the liver tissue resulting in cellular death hardening and the formation of scar tissue. Thiamine, responsible for the health of the nervous system, is also largely destroyed by alcohol [2]. This results in a lack of appetite and arrested growth as well as weight loss. Over the longer term thiamine deficiency leads to Wernicke's encephalopathy, which consists of disorientation and dementia due to the irreversible neuronal damage done by alcoholic destruction of thiamine [2]. Other neurological effects of alcohol found predominantly in adolescents are impaired verbal learning and cognitive development; this effect is aggravated by concomitant use of marijuana [17].

Of major concern is the role of alcohol consumption in type 2 adult onset diabetes, which is globally on the rise. The incidence of this widespread problem was lower in former years in the Far East; however, the trend today is for the populations in countries such as Japan to be as much at risk as those in the Westernised world. Research has shown a direct link between alcohol consumption and type 2 diabetes [18]. Chronic heavy drinking patterns and acute or long-term alcohol dependency carries risks that may not always be calculated into the health care burden. Recent findings have shown that alcoholic patients have a three to fourfold increase in the development of severe postoperative infection and toxic shock over those who are non-drinkers [19].

'Alcohol relatedness' varies across diseases. This is commonly expressed in 'alcohol attributable fractions' (AAF). Some diseases or consequences are fully attributable to alcohol (e.g. the alcohol dependence syndrome), other consequences have a high alcohol attribution such as liver cirrhosis, for some consequences there are many other factors which may cause a disease, among which alcohol often plays one role, and thus the alcohol attributable part may be low [16]. Alcohol consumption during pregnancy is also of concern because there is no established safe limit; women who are pregnant or planning pregnancy are advised to avoid alcohol completely. Excessive alcohol during pregnancy is a recognised cause of developmental delays known as foetal alcohol syndrome (FAS) and foetal alcohol effects [20]. Officially FAS affects one in 1000 live births of infants and has broad health and social consequences [20]. The reality is that more children are entering school with FAS-related learning difficulties and presenting at health centres with symptoms of FAS, suggesting that the problem is underreported [20]. Even children less visibly affected by FAS and for whom the problem may have gone unnoticed, have been found to be a greater risk of behavioural problems [21]. The teratogenic (pre-natal damage) effects of alcohol appear to lie across a spectrum, in which damage may be mild to severe, depending on consumption and the ability of the mother to metabolise alcohol, however, there appears to be no place on the spectrum of consumption of alcohol during pregnancy where there will be no consequences [21].

Quick Quiz

1. The two nutrients that are most likely to be destroyed by alcohol consumption are:

Answer: _____

A. Magnesium and Thiamine

B. Riboflavin and Potassium

C. Iron and Vitamin A

D. Vitamin C and Sodium

2. The destruction or lack of enzymes needed for metabolism is caused by the alcoholic destruction of:

Answer: _____

A. Thiamine

B. Magnesium

C. Acetaldehyde

D. Antabuse

3. The hardening of the liver due to alcohol consumption is known as

Answer: _____

A. Cirrhosis

B. Wernicke's Syndrome

C. Foetal Alcohol Syndrome

D. Adult onset Type 2 Diabetes

4. The percentage of drinkers who are likely to become dependent on alcohol is approximately:

Answer: _____

A. 2%

B. 5%

C. 10%

D. 25%

5. Women who are pregnant or planning pregnancy are advised to:

Answer: _____

A. Consume less than 5 drinks at once

B. Consume less than 5 drinks per week

C. Spread their drinks out during the week

D. Not consume any alcohol

How Much is Enough and How Much is Too Much?

There have been some controversial and confounding results of research into the effects of alcohol on the cardiovascular system. In older studies on alcohol use, both good and adverse effects have been noted [22]. Studies have found that even light to moderate consumption of alcohol (more than 2 drinks per week) can increase blood pressure in inactive desk-bound men [22]. It has been found that the increase is directly related to the amount of alcohol drunk and that the difference in health between drinkers and non-drinkers is greater in those aged 35 and over [22].

Small benefits to the cardiovascular system have previously been found with moderate consumption of alcohol [23], predominantly red wine. The benefit has been found to be the result of the flavonoid content of red and black grapes on the platelet aggravating factors and blood lipid profile (the amount of fat in the blood and its level of 'stickiness') [23]. The same amount of flavonoid content as has been found in red wine will be found in the same volume of red grape juice. In addition, resveratrol found in grapes independently reduces not only the risk of heart disease and other inflammatory conditions but also the risk of certain cancers [24-25]. Consuming red or black grapes, red or blackcurrants, red plums, raspberries and blackberries will also have a beneficial effect on heart health. The most recent studies have found that there are no benefits whatsoever to alcohol consumption and any benefit arising out of particular alcoholic drinks may be due to factors other than the alcoholic content [26]

The overall volume of alcohol consumed is probably the most important causative factor in the generation of chronic health disorders such as cirrhosis of the liver [27]. When viewing the consumption of alcohol as a causative factor in accidental deaths and sociological problems, however, it is the individual episodes of heavy drinking alongside the context in which this drinking takes place which is of concern [16, 27]. Alcohol consumption varies between countries and cultures; however, statistically, women are more likely to be lifetime abstainers than men and persons who reside in areas where the dominant religion is Islam are likely to abstain from alcohol regardless of whether they practice this religion or not [16]. Conversely, it is mainly men who are the heaviest drinkers as opposed to women who, almost across the board, consume far less alcohol [16].

There is widespread agreement that the health and well-being of many young people today are seriously being threatened using alcohol. Worries have arisen internationally, as emerging trends in consumption are starting to permeate youth culture, across the board, transcending national boundaries. Drinking in high school leads to drinking in college or university, and there is a tendency to overestimate how much alcohol intake is 'normal' in the social context [28]. These trends have revealed a more hedonistic attitude towards continuous drinking, binge drinking and frequent intoxication, purely for the psychologically pleasurable experience [28]. Going out with friends for the sole purpose of getting drunk is increasingly viewed in a positive light amongst those in the 18-24 year age group [28].

The Tenth Revision of the International Classification of Diseases and Health Problems (ICD-10) defines alcohol dependence syndrome as: 'a cluster of physiological, behavioural, and cognitive phenomena in which the use of alcohol takes on a much higher priority for a given individual than other behaviours that once had greater value'. This is often viewed as a very strong or even compulsive and overpowering desire for alcohol with total disregard both for other needs and the consequences of drinking [16].

Restrictions on the sale of alcohol, including curtailing the days, times, density and places of sales, limits the possibilities of consumers to buy and consume alcoholic beverages. This may reduce overall and heavy alcohol consumption. It has been found that curbing the number of alcoholic beverage outlets and regulating their location has a significant effect on sales of alcohol. Conversely, the geographical placement of outlets that sell alcohol and a heavier concentration of such outlets in certain areas is associated with an increase in alcohol-related problems, such as violence and drunk driving [29].

Overall, researchers share the view that there is no reason for abstainers from alcohol to start drinking or for those who occasionally drink to increase their consumption to obtain health benefits [30]. There are many other things that one can do to obtain the same health benefits, such as attention to diet, especially to fruit and vegetable consumption, and regular cardiovascular exercise [30]. With rising rates of alcohol consumption and extensive high-risk drinking, both chronic and acute damage from alcohol is expected to increase [27] Attention is needed to [31]:

- o create effective policies and interventions;
- o control access to alcohol;
- o reduce high-risk drinking; and
- o provide brief interventions for high-risk drinkers

Learning Together

Activity 4.2: Take approximately 15 minutes for this activity.

In small groups, take one of the following issues:

a). The cardioprotective or other health benefits of the resveratrol content of alcohol vs the possible increase in blood pressure;

b). The health benefits of relaxation and lowering of inhibitions vs the possible risks (i.e. incapacitated rape and drunk driving);

c). The cost of drinking to the employer, health care institutions and increase in social problems and crime vs the government tax benefit and the money made by the industry or;

d). The social benefits of alcohol such as going out with friends and traditional celebrations such as weddings and birthdays vs the social costs of crime, road accidents and violence.

On balance:

1. What benefits outweigh the possible consequences of alcohol consumption in the chosen argument?

2. What protective factors could be implemented to counteract the risks from alcohol consumption?

Your answers and opinions may be brought into the discussion we are about to have.

Group Discussion

SOMETHING IS NOT WORKING WITH ALCOHOL SALES AND CONSUMPTION OR IS NOW THE TIME FOR A RETHINK?

In light of the above research and the growing admission of many countries as well as individuals to the problems of alcohol consumption, alcohol use is now under heavy debate. Even the WHO has issued a report on alcohol that is as pressing as reports on nutrition, HIV/AIDS and infectious disease. Despite the age-old relationship with alcohol in the form of a safe and convenient beverage in times when water was not fit for consumption to the recent scourge of death on the roads, we have come to the point where decisions need to be made on a global level. We ask ourselves in this discussion:

- Firstly, what are the benefits that we can see from the consumption of alcohol that cannot be gained by other means?
- The hospitality industry focusses on those who consume alcohol, either in food or in hotel-room bar fridges, and bar lounges. Yet, at least one-third of the world's population does not drink, either for religious, health or social reasons. On balance, do you think that the industry caters rightly for the majority or that they lose out from those who choose not to consume alcohol?
- What measures do you as a group think could be implemented with respect to the control and sale of alcohol:
    - At present?
    - In the future?

References

1. Drope, J.; Schluger, N.; Cahn, Z.; Drope J; Hamil, S.; Islami, F.; Liber, A.; Nargis, N.; Stoklosa, M., *The Tobacco Atlas*. 6 ed.; The American Cancer Society: Atlanta, USA, 2018.

2. Sackheim, G. L.; Lehman, D. D., *Chemistry for the Health Sciences*. 2nd ed.; Macmillan: New York, 1994.

3. Clark, N. M.; Baily, W. C.; Rand, C., Advances in Prevention and Education in Lung Disease. *American Journal of Respiratory Critical Care Medicine* **1998,** (157), S155-S167.

4. Mackay, J.; Erikson, M.; Shafey, O., The Tobacco Atlas. 2 ed.; American Cancer Society: Atlanta USA, 2006. (accessed November 2006).

5. Pednekar, M. S.; Gupta, P. C.; Shukla, H. C.; Hebert, J. R. Association between tobacco use and body mass index in urban Indian population: Implications for public health in India *Biomed Central: Public Health* [Online], 2006. http://www.biomedcentral.com/1471-2458/6/70.

6. World Health Organisation *WHO Report on the Global Tobacco Epidemic, 2011: Warning about the dangers of tobacco*; World Health Organisation: Geneva, 2011.

7. Persaud, R., *The Mind*. Bantam Press: London, 2007.

8. Lee, K.; Collin, J. "Key to the Future": British American Tobacco and Cigarette Smuggling in China *PLoS Medicine* [Online], 2006, p. 1080-1089. http//www.plosmedicine.org (accessed 5th September 2008).

9. Nowak, T. J.; Handford, A. G., *Pathophysiology: Concepts and Applications for Health Care Professionals*. 3rd ed.; McGraw-Hill: New York, 2004.

10. Larsen, S.; Haavaldsen, C.; Bjelland, E. K.; Dypvik, J.; Jukic, A. M.; Eskild, A., Placental weight and birthweight: the relations with number of daily cigarettes and smoking cessation in pregnancy. A population study. *Int J Epidemiol* **2018,** *47* (4), 1141-1150.

11. Scott, J. G.; Matuschka, L.; Niemela, S.; Miettunen, J.; Emmerson, B.; Mustonen, A., Evidence of a Causal Relationship Between Smoking Tobacco and Schizophrenia Spectrum Disorders. *Front Psychiatry* **2018,** *9*, 607.

12. Bertuccio, P.; La Vecchia, C.; Silverman, D. T.; Petersen, G. M.; M, B. P.; Negri, E.; Li, D.; Risch, H. A.; Olson, S. H.; Gallinger, S.; Miller, A. B.; Bueno-de-Mesquita, H. B.; Talamini, R.; Polesel, J.; Ghadirian, P.; Baghurst, P. A.; Zatonski, W.; Fontham, E. T.; Bamlet, W. R.; Holly, E. A.; Lucenteforte, E.; Hassan, M.; Yu, H.; Kurtz, R. C.; Cotterchio, M.; Su, J.; Maisonneuve, P.; Duell, E. J.; Bosetti, C.; Boffetta, P. Cigar and pipe smoking, smokeless tobacco use and pancreatic cancer: an analysis from the International Pancreatic Cancer Case-Control Consortium (PanC4) *Annals of oncology :* p. 1420-1426. (accessed 6 September 2012).

13. Mejia, A. B.; Ling, P. M.; Glantz, S. A. Quantifying the effects of promoting smokeless tobacco as a harm reduction strategy in the USA *Tobacco control* [Online], 2010, p. 297-305. (accessed 6 September 2012).

14. Earl, R., Guidelines for Dietary Planning. In *Krause's Food Nutrition and Diet Therapy*, 11th ed.; Mahan, L. K.; Escott-Stump, S., Eds. Saunders Elsevier: Philadelphia, 2004.

15. The Guardian Newspaper Child Labour Rampant in Tobacco Industry. http://tmssmagazine. com/child-labour-rampant-in-tobacco-industry/ (accessed 23 March 2018).

16. WHO *Global Status Report on Alcohol*; World Health Organisation: Geneva, Switzerland, 2004.

17. Medina, K. L.; Nagel, B. J.; Park, A.; McQueeny, T.; Tapert, S. F., Depressive symptoms in adolescents: associations with white matter volume and marijuana use. *Journal of Child Psychology and Psychiatry* **2007,** *48* (6), 592-600.

18. Waki, K.; Noda, M.; Sasaki, S.; Matsumura, Y.; Takahashi, Y.; Isogawa, A.; Ohashi, Y.; Kadowaki, T.; Tsugane, S., Alcohol consumption and other risk factors for self-reported diabetes among middle-aged Japanese: a population-based prospective study in the JPHC study cohort I. *Diabetic medicine : a journal of the British Diabetic Association* **2005,** *22* (3), 323-31.

19. von Dossow, V.; Schilling, C.; Beller, S.; Vargas Hein, O.; von Heymann, C.; Kox, W. J.; Spies, C. D. Altered immune parameters in chronic alcoholic patients at the onset of infection and of septic shock *Critical Care* [Online], 2004, p. R312-R321. http://ccforum. com/content/8/5/R312 (accessed 22nd March 2007).

20. Morleo, M.; Woolfall, K.; Dedman, D.; Mukherjee, R.; Bellis, M. A.; Cook, P. A. Under-reporting of foetal alcohol spectrum disorders: an analysis of hospital episode statistics *Biomed Central Pediatrics* [Online], 2011. http://www.biomedcentral.com/1471-2431/11/14 (accessed 10 September 2012).

21. Fagerlund, Å.; Autti-Rämö, I.; Hoyme, H. E.; Mattson, S. N.; Korkman, M. Risk factors for behavioural problems in foetal alcohol spectrum disorders *Acta Paediatrica* [Online], 2011, p. 1481-1488. (accessed 10 September 2012).

22. Nakanishi, N.; Makino, K.; Nishina, K.; Suzuki, K.; Tatara, K. Relationship of Light to Moderate Alcohol Consumption and Risk of Hypertension in Japanese Male Office Workers *Alcoholism: Clinical and Environmental Research* [Online], 2002, p. 988-994. (accessed 15 November 2006).

23. de Lorgeril, M.; Salen, P. Is alcohol anti-inflammatory in the context of coronary heart disease? *Heart* [Online], 2004, p. 355-357. http://www.heartjnl.com (accessed 23rd August 2007).

24. Lomholt, S.; Mellemkjaer, A.; Iversen, M. B.; Pedersen, S. B.; Kragstrup, T. W., Resveratrol displays anti-inflammatory properties in an ex vivo model of immune-mediated inflammatory arthritis. *BMC Rheumatol* **2018,** *2*, 27.

25. Yang, Z.; Xie, Q.; Chen, Z.; Ni, H.; Xia, L.; Zhao, Q.; Chen, Z.; Chen, P., Resveratrol suppresses the invasion and migration of human gastric cancer cells via inhibition of MALAT1-mediated epithelial-to-mesenchymal transition. *Exp Ther Med* **2019,** *17* (3), 1569-1578.

26. Burton, R.; Sheron, N. No level of alcohol consumption improves health *The Lancet* [Online], 2018. https://doi.org/10.1016/S0140-6736(18)31571-X (accessed 30 August 2018).

27. Yokoyama, H., Relationship Between Ethanol Consumption Level and Lifestyle Status: Excessive Ethanol Consumption Can Account for the Prevalence of Lifestyle-Related Diseases. *Alcoholism Clinical and Experimental Research* **2005,** *29* (12), 294-297.

28. Beck, K. H.; Arria, A. M.; Caldeira, K. M.; Vincent, K. B.; O'Grady, K. E.; Wish, E. D., Social context of drinking and alcohol problems among college students. *American Journal of Health Behaviour* **2008,** *32* (4), 420-430.

29. WHO *Global Status Report: Alcohol Policy*; World Health Organisation: Geneva, Switzerland, 2004.

30. Walker, J. M.; Eckardt, P.; Aleman, J. O.; da Rosa, J. C.; Liang, Y.; Iizumi, T.; Etheve, S.; Blaser, M. J.; J, L. B.; Holt, P. R., The effects of trans-resveratrol on insulin resistance, inflammation, and microbiota in men with the metabolic syndrome: A pilot randomized, placebo-controlled clinical trial. *J Clin Transl Res* **2019,** *4* (2), 122-135.

31. Rehm, J.; Giesbrecht, N.; Patra, J.; Roerecke, M. Estimating Chronic Disease Deaths and Hospitalizations Due to Alcohol Use in Canada in 2002: Implications for Policy and Prevention Strategies *Preventing Chronic Disease* [Online], 2006. http://www.cdc.gov/pcd/issues2006/oct/05-0009.htm (accessed 22nd March 2007).

LEARNING SESSION FIVE: PILLS AND POTIONS – THE RIGHT WAY AND THE WRONG WAY TO USE MEDICATION

Introduction

In this session, we look at the definition of medicine, and what types of medicines are available. We review the correct way to use medication and how to seek professional health care advice. We discuss what you can do for yourself and when it is appropriate to ask for assistance. We also look at the question of who to ask for assistance, health care qualifications, and professional registration being essential to correct service delivery of treatment. In turn, when we receive a prescription, we should follow through with the correct procedure. Antibiotics are lifesavers and have drastically reduced the death toll from some previously untreatable problems; however, they have become over-used over the years. We discuss the appropriate use and possible abuse of antibiotics, painkillers and over the counter remedies as well as commonly used complementary medicines and how to understand and adhere to instructions. At this stage, we come to our first learning together session, where we look at what should be included in a set of instructions.

We then move on to the globally growing problem of recreational substance abuse as well as addiction, not only to illegal drugs but also to over the counter and prescribed medications. What has fuelled this self-medication trend and are we solving anything by attempting to treat ourselves, or are we compounding the problems? In our second learning together session, we look at what one wants from a practitioner, is it always medication? If so, for how long should a substance, even if it is a 'legal' one, be prescribed? We then come to our discussion for the day, which focuses on internet medicine sales. Many of these are for so-called life enhancers and offer smart pills, slimming pills and cosmetic aids over the 'net'; are they genuine or are they playing on the 'fear factor' that people have regarding possible social unacceptability and failure?

Ice-Breaker Quiz

True / False

1. If you are prescribed an antibiotic you should stop taking them immediately you start to feel better

_____

2. The maximum number of over the counter pain killer tablets you can take in one day is 20

_____

3. Grapefruit and grapefruit juice can interact with prescribed and over the counter medications

_____

4. Antibiotics are used to treat viral conditions

_____

5. It is best to wait until you have a disease before you receive a vaccination for it

_____

6. Cough and cold medications can keep you awake at night

_____

7. If your medicine has been prescribed by a doctor there is no need for you to read the package insert

_____

8. Once you have finished a medicine it is best to get another prescription to prevent the problem recurring

_____

9. The main ingredient in many cough mixtures is alcohol

_____

10. Taking pain medication in advance will prevent stress induced headaches

_____

What Constitutes a 'Medicine'?

Technically a medicine is a drug or any other substance taken to treat or prevent disease [1]. There is no technical distinction between pharmaceutical medications and natural, herbal or home preparations, although the term is generally used in most developed countries to describe pharmaceutical substances. For many people in both developing countries, and some in developed countries, the traditional use of herbal preparations and traditional healing methods continues in many cases alongside the more modern use of pharmacology [2]. There are medicines that kill and those that save, some that cause adverse side effects and some that take away most of life's discomforts; there are those that create problems and those that prevent them, some medicines work, and some do not [3-4].

The total number of prescription drugs, as well as the overall quantities taken by consumers, has skyrocketed in recent years and in some areas has become a cause for concern [5-7]. The potential for correct use of ethically and professionally prescribed pharmaceutical medicines for better quality and longer life cannot be disputed; however, along with benefits, there are considerations [5-7]. The downside is that inappropriate, excessive, careless and less than optimal prescribing of medications can become a silent killer [6]. While some people in the developing world are at risk from inadequate medication, some in the developed world are at risk from iatrogenic diseases caused by overmedication or multiple drug interactions [6].

Traditional medicine (TM) is a comprehensive term used to refer both to systems such as traditional Chinese medicine, Indian Ayurveda and Arabic Unani-Tibb medicine, and to various forms of indigenous medicine. In countries where the dominant health care system is based on allopathic medicine, or where TM has not been incorporated into the national health care system, TM is often termed "complementary", "alternative" or "non-conventional" medicine [8]. The spectrum of medicines that indigenous traditional healers, as well as well-respected professional medical systems of healing, such as ayurvedic, traditional Chinese and Unani-Tibb uses, includes foods, leaves, flowers and roots of plants, animal matter and mineral compounds, which in many cases appears to have a long history of safe and effective use [8]. Despite this, traditional drugs and traditional medicine in general, represent a still poorly explored field of research in terms of therapeutic potential or clinical evaluation. There is a current preoccupation about this since it is well-established that all sorts of vegetable, animal and mineral remedies used in a traditional setting are capable of producing serious adverse reactions [8].

Currently, 75% of the global population uses traditional or unconventional medicine to some degree, and for many in developing countries it is the main source of medical assistance, and by default, the 'norm' in the use of medicines [2]. It is essential, however, that traditional drug therapies be subject to appropriate risk to benefit analysis both to preserve the use of those that are potentially of global benefit as well as to curtail their inappropriate or unsafe use [8]. In addition, the monitoring and control of the use of safe and effective traditional medicines are required in order to foster their use within the framework of public health [8].

Aside from this, there is the controversial use of nutritional substances. The prescribed use of these, alongside an individualised dietary regime, is termed 'nutritional medicine' [9]. The argument for the use of nutritional supplements is that this cannot be separated out from concomitant dietary intervention and both modalities are required. If no overt claims are made for such a substance, it may not fall under any legal control and is therefore freely available. There is considerable debate over whether such substances are deemed to be medicinal. The substances prescribed are often available without recourse to professional consultation, and there is the possibility of self-medicating to one's personal detriment, a situation no different essentially from that of self-medicating with over the counter pharmaceutical substances.

When to Get Help and Where to Get Help

No-one can argue against prevention being better than cure, and many disorders are connected to lifestyle, however, when illness and discomfort arises, there is a need for the alleviation of pain and discomfort at the very least. The concept of equity of access to health care is a central objective of many health care systems and has been an important buttress of the UK and other National Health Services [10]. Yet the concept nevertheless remains somewhat elusive, and research evidence on the nature and magnitude of inequities, although extensive, proves patchy and difficult to interpret [10]. As a result, it is often not straightforward to decide whether inequities in access pose a significant policy problem and if so, how they might best be tackled [10]. The reality is that many people view professional help as expensive, time consuming and unnecessary and, even if it is free at source, appointments might be difficult to obtain within a reasonable time.

The first recourse is always prevention, and simple non-intervention techniques are often helpful in alleviating minor problems such as minor gastric upsets, stress-induced headaches and fatigue. Some of these include the following [11].

- Adequate intake of fluid, especially plain clear water from a safe drinking source
- Adequate sleep
- A short walk in the fresh air
- A good, well-balanced diet and, if experiencing a minor gastric upset, plain un-spiced foods or the BRAT diet (bananas, rice, cooked apple and plain dry whole-wheat toast)

Should these measures not suffice to alleviate the problem, one may require medication or further assistance. Taking medicine, however, is not something that one should ever do without advice from a professionally qualified person. This is especially true if one is already taking some form of medication for a chronic problem on a long-term basis and a further problem occurs, an infection develops, or you have an accident or injury [12]. The question of when to get help is an easy one to answer; it is almost always. Apart from minor injuries such as cuts and scrapes, extensive injuries, uncontrolled or prolonged bleeding and any adverse symptoms of illness that prevent one from going to school or work requires professional advice. Certainly, it would be advisable to seek advice should any of the following occur:

- Persistent nausea, vomiting if occurring for more than one hour and especially if accompanied by headache, dizziness, abdominal pain or swelling
- Persistent changes in bowel habits, especially if accompanied by pain, swelling or bleeding
- Any incidence of fainting, loss of consciousness or dizziness accompanied by changes in sight and/or hearing
- Untoward bleeding of any nature that does not abate of its own accord within 30 minutes (i.e. persistent nose bleeds, moles or scars that begin to bleed).
- Pain and / or bruising and / or swelling that cannot be explained by a recent minor injury
- Sudden weight loss not due to dieting, especially if accompanied by extreme thirst, dizziness, changes in sight.
- Frequent urination, especially if accompanied by cloudy or burning urine
- Fever or temperature accompanied by excessive perspiration
- Restricted ability to breathe, breathlessness upon exertion, especially if accompanied by chest pain
- Intermittent chest pain, upper abdominal pain, heartburn or indigestion which recurs and/or persists
- Painful swollen joints, especially if accompanied by changes in body temperature.
- Upper respiratory tract discomfort such as persistent sore throat, difficulty in swallowing, earache, persistent nasal congestion, especially if accompanied by headache
- Swollen glands behind the ears, knees and in the groin, which are painful to touch

In the first instance, it would be best to seek the advice of an integrated health care practitioner if such a service is available to you. Failing this, one's first recourse for a minor problem would be a qualified pharmacist who would be able to ascertain whether an over the counter pharmaceutical, herbal or nutritional product might solve the problem. In addition, your regular pharmacist is likely to be aware of any medication that you are currently using and of any possible interaction between your regular medication and anything else that you might use on a temporary basis [13]. Should your regular pharmacist not be able to offer any assistance or recommend that you seek further professional help, you have the option of seeking out the kind of assistance that is acceptable to you. This may be a general medical practitioner, certified health consultant, or someone with a more specific and specialist orientation such as a chiropractor, dietician, physiotherapist or counsellor. Regardless of the type of person you see, the following guidelines are to be recommended with respect to the health care professional with whom you consult [13-14]

- They have the qualifications that match the type of assistance you are seeking and that these qualifications are either displayed in the practice or are verifiable
- That they are registered with a professional body which has an enforceable code of ethics
- That they operate within the boundaries of their ability and are prepared to refer you to someone else should they or you, require further assistance
- They can see you within a reasonable amount of time before the problem is likely to worsen

Quick Quiz

Using coloured pens or pencils match up the health care problem in the left column with the type of health care practitioner in the right column that you think you should consult (there may be more than one possibility).

1. Your eyesight is becoming blurred and you are having difficulty reading the small print, you get a headache after reading for a while

A. General Practitioner

2. You are suddenly putting on a lot of weight for no apparent reason and wish to lose it

B. Nutritionist

C. Naturopath

3. You have suddenly lost a lot of weight, are feeling tired, run down and generally unwell

D. Optometrist

4. You are having a lot of headaches which are gradually becoming worse, you have developed thread veins on your face and are having a problem managing your stressful job

E. Physiotherapist

F. Personal Trainer

G. Counsellor

5. You have been having indigestion type pain for a while on and off but now it seems to be occurring almost every day, especially if you exert yourself Therapist

H. Chiropractor

I. Stress Management

6. You are overweight, almost always tired and your back, knees and ankles are beginning to ache, especially when you have to walk somewhere or carry heavy shopping

Correct Use of Medication: Understanding and Following Directions

Drug resistance has been an ongoing problem for decades and is of increasing international concern [15]. Bacteria often live in harmony with other inhabitants of the Earth. Since penicillin, however, became widely available in 1942, and other antibiotics soon followed, the killing and growth-inhibitory effects of antibiotics have applied selective pressure that has reduced the number of susceptible strains, leading to the propagation of more resistant varieties of bacteria. The selection and spread of these varieties are facilitated paradoxically by either over-prescribing or under-prescribing of drugs [16]. Resistance genes continue to be selected in malaria organisms causing resurgences in disease incidence. The international spread of multiple-drug-resistant malaria organisms in Southeast Asia has been attributed largely to movements of civilians during civil disturbances [15].

Inappropriate use of antibiotics is common in primary care, and effective interventions are needed to promote judicious antibiotic use and reduce antibiotic resistance [17]. In addition, intermittent and interrupted use of tuberculosis medication has created a global problem in increasing the strains of drug-resistant tuberculosis [18]. When taking either antibiotics or tuberculosis medication, it is important to remember the following:

- Take the medication daily as recommended, do not skip doses or take fewer tablets or take them less often for them to last longer.
- Do not stop taking the medication in the middle of the treatment, take all the tablets / capsules / powders you have been given.
- If the problem is still there on the last day of medication, contact your GP, or pharmacist, clinic or hospital outpatient nurse for advice, you may need more medication, a stronger dose or different medication.
- If the side effects of medication are so extreme, such as acute gastrointestinal distress, vomiting, or dizziness, contact someone immediately (even if it is the emergency centre) before stopping the medication. It is possible that the medication may have to be changed.

Many persons live with a chronic disorder today that they would not have lived with as little as twenty years ago. Increasing numbers of people are becoming life-long users of some form of medication and as many as 40% of those who are, use medication for more than one chronic problem [12]. Understanding the management of the medication they use, avoiding side effects and interactions is important to the quality of life of persons in this category. There may, however, be barriers to achieving this finely tuned balance between the intended good health management. For some, this includes increasing age and deteriorating levels of cognition, for others the complexity of following different regimens for a number of different medications [12]. Effective management of chronic illness is complex and requires significant participation by patients and their families. Day-to-day disease self-management has multiple components [12]:

- Engaging in activities that promote physical and psychological health;
- Monitoring health status and making associated care decisions;
- Managing the impact of the illness on physical, psychological and social functioning
- Interacting with health care providers and adherence to treatment recommendations. This will also mean that the following guidelines need to be noted:
    - If you do not understand the instructions for taking medication or are not sure what the side effects may be, then you must ask
    - If the instructions are not in your home language / language of use, then ask someone who speaks your language to explain the instructions to you and make your own notes
    - Make sure that you know whether to take each of your medications with or without food, before or after a meal
    - Make sure that you are clear about whether the treatment will be short, medium or long term and whether you will require repeat prescriptions for medication.
    - Make sure that you are clear about further consultations, where to go and who to contact.

In addition to the problems experienced by inappropriate or over-prescribed medication are those of self-medication and use of over the counter preparations that also fall under the term 'medicine'. Often, no professional help has been sought regarding their use. The type of medicines sold without a prescription varies greatly and depends upon local pharmaceutical laws as well as control and monitoring mechanisms in place.

In the UK, an estimated 59% of the population and 44% of the population in the US appear to be regular users of herbal medications and nutritional supplements [13]. Over the counter, herbal preparations are also used not only by relatively healthy persons for minor ailments or general health and well-being but also by those who have long term chronic disorders, pregnant and breastfeeding women, children and the elderly [13]. As with conventional medicines, it is reasonable to expect that there will be some interaction between conventional medications taken on a regular basis and herbal medications taken without advice [13]. Concerns with regard to the concurrent use of pharmaceutical and non-allopathic medications are amplified when the health care consumer does not take professional advice with regard to their decisions, especially when the fear of disapproval either by the conventional or non-allopathic practitioner drives a lack of disclosure [13]. It is appropriate to remember that the ultimate choice is in the hands of the health care consumer and, if personal choices are being undermined, one is at liberty to find someone with a more integrated and holistic approach to health and well-being.

Learning Together

Activity 5.1: Allow approximately 20 minutes for this exercise.

Below we are going to look at items that may or may not be on the package insert for prescribed or over the counter medicines. We ask you to pick the five items that your group think would be the most important information for the person who is taking the medication.

What time of day to take the medicine
How often it can be taken
Whether or not one should take it before, with or after food
For how long it is safe to take the medicine
Which company manufactured the medicine
Who to write to if you have a complaint
The 'sell by / use by' date
Who the medicine is safe for
Who should not take the medicine
What to do if you are not getting any better
How to get a discount
Where to buy more medicine if you need it
What to do if you experience an adverse effect from the medicine
What other products the manufacturer makes
Whether free samples of the medicine are available

The most important items to include are:

1. _____

2. _____

3. _____

4. _____

5. _____

Which of the above does your group feel is the most important and why?

_____
_____
_____

You may now like to take five minutes to discuss these answers.

Compounding the Problems: Illegal Substances, Recreational and Inappropriate Use

At its origin, the definition of an addiction is a 'giving-over' or ' engaging in a behaviour habitually' with either positive or negative implications [19]. More recently this has come to mean a strong overpowering urge to engage in either a behaviour or intake of a substance to one's detriment [19]. Addictions can come in many forms including addictive behaviours involving excessive cell-phone or computer use, gaming and gambling, as well as the use of certain foods, alcohol and both legal and illegal pharmaceutical substances [19]. It is the latter with which we are concerned in this session.

The prevalence of addictions in the US has been reported to be approximately 47% [20]. Globally, cannabis is the most commonly used illegal drug in Westernised societies, with almost one-third of fifteen-year-olds having used this substance [21]. The main psychoactive ingredient targets the pleasure / reward system in the brain, producing endogenous chemicals in the brain (endocannabinoids) that induce temporary feelings of well-being and happiness [21], however, there is a debilitating after effect. Cannabis use amongst teenagers appears to predispose users to depression and anxiety, in a dose / use-dependent manner with frequent users developing an increasing tendency towards depression and anxiety disorders during adult life [21]. Unfortunately, almost one-third of cannabis users (approximately 15% of teenagers) in this society are likely to progress on to other more addictive substances including Class A drugs such as injectable amphetamines, ecstasy and cocaine [21].

MDMA / ecstasy, LSD, amphetamines and GHB are commonly used 'club drugs' [22]. The use of these too is increasing globally, and there are serious concerns in the medical profession, not only about the short term consequences but the long term problem of immune suppression, which has now come to light [23]. MDMA / ecstasy is of particular concern as this drug suppresses the same CD4-T cells as the HIV virus [23]. The use of 'club drugs' is also likely to increase during holidays away from home and short overseas working breaks and is more likely to reflect the use of drugs in the holiday environment than that in the home community [24]. Use of drugs while on longer holidays and extended visits is also likely to increase when the traveller is male and without a partner or spouse [24]. As many of these drugs increase the risk of microbial infections, their use places an increased burden upon the health care community in countries hosting young tourists as well as an additional financial burden on insurers and users alike [24].

A recent survey in the US found that teenagers and those in their early twenties are more likely to be multiple drug users than older adults and to use a combination of drugs and alcohol [22]. This type of problem brings with it far greater risks of overdose, cardiac failure and drug-induced multiple organ failure and / or coma and death and is of major concern amongst the health care professionals that deal with such medical crises [22]. Equally disconcerting is the fact that less than 1% of 'club drug' users stay with this class of drugs or use them only for occasional social use [22].

Most socially abused drugs target the endocannabinoid system that produces similar feelings of reward and happiness, [21] the differences being only in the intensity, duration and time elapsed. Hence targeting this neurological system with a blocking agent that prevents the endogenous production of endocannabinoids substances might hold some promise for treating addictive disorders in the future [21]. In the meantime, researchers found that those who remain in school, are married and / or have stable family relationships are less likely to use drugs and are also less likely to engage in other risky behaviours [22].

Some substances that are habit-forming may, in fact, be legal or were once bona-fide over the counter (OTC) medications or nutritional supplements. Such was the case with GHB and its derivative gamma-butyrolactone (GABA), a significantly new substance that has been added to the list of controlled substances in the US since 2000 [25]. The claims made by supplement companies who have marketed GABA are that it enhances lean muscle growth, aids sleep and improves sexual performance [25]. Use of this substance with alcohol commonly produces nausea and vomiting but can induce coma and death [25].

Pain killers may be both under and over-used in many instances [26-27]. Fear of inducing tolerance and confusion of tolerance with addiction, as well as the possibility of attracting addicts to one's practice, are amongst the most common fears that practitioners have with respect to prescribing opiates for chronic long-term pain [28]. This reluctance to prescribe moderate use of more effective drugs may drive patients into the chronic over-use of over the counter painkillers. Even when initially correctly prescribed, prescription drugs are not problem free. It is estimated that 8 million US Citizens are using prescription drugs for longer than recommended or for problems that are best solved by other means [29]. Of these, 1.3 million people in the US, aged 12 years and over are actively abusing prescription drugs, painkillers (analgesics) being the most widely abused [29].

Self-medication has, in some instances, been fuelled by mistrust, practitioner overload and the patient's perception of being treated inappropriately by conventional practitioners [30]. More than 20% of the UK population has at some point in time accessed non-conventional healthcare either seeking out an alternative or traditional practitioner or using over the counter supplements, herbs and other items [30]. Most practitioners' welcome the patients' input into their own health and encourage greater self-responsibility and patient participation in the decision making with regard to long term health and well-being [30]. This is, however, with the proviso that the correct health care is sought and advice is taken appropriately, even with non-conventional care [30].

Learning Together

Activity 5.2: Allow approximately 20 minutes for this exercise

In small learning groups look at the following suggestions given for what you may or may not receive from a health care visit and decide between you which are the five most important things that you would like to come away with.

A prescription for initial medication
Onward referral to a consultant
Advice as to what I can do for myself to alleviate the problem
Advice about diet
Herbal or other natural medication
Some form of testing to ascertain what is wrong
A diagnosis of what the problem is
An explanation of why I have the problem that I have
Advice about where I can get further information about my problem
Referral to a support group or patient association
A prescription that they can repeat or that lasts a good six months
Medication that I can take for the rest of my life

The most important items to include are:

1. _____

2. _____

3. _____

4. _____

5. _____

Which of the above does your group feel is the most important and why?

_____

_____

_____

You may now like to take five minutes to discuss these answers.

Group Discussion

INTERNET SALES OF PHARMACEUTICAL 'LIFE ENHANCERS' FLOGGING THE 'FEAR FACTOR'!

GABA discussed in the previous section is still available over the internet and is marketed as a dietary supplement that helps you cut fat and build lean muscle tissue. Hoodia, a herbal substance is recommended for cutting appetite and slimming is also one of many slimming aids available over the internet in various doses without dietary advice being given or the problem of why one is obese being addressed. 'Smart Pills' have also become popular as have those that keep you awake and alert, ostensibly to get more done in the day and become more successful. Viagra and Cialis are not only available as sex aids over the internet from pharmaceutical dealers but are often offered in unsolicited e-mails that go out to millions of e-mail users daily, all over the world. Many of these dealers operate from developing countries, illegally, where there is little likelihood of their being controlled, regulated or in any way checked on by government agencies. These services are increasing because they are used, and this type of pharmaceutical sale is obviously profitable, but why? We ask ourselves in this discussion: Is this a genuine service and representative of the publics' freedom to choose, or do these businesses play on the fact that obesity, academic and career competitiveness and a flagging sex life are sources of embarrassment? Hence, the growth of the self-medication market!

- Do you think that buying pills for your problems over the internet is a good way to save money and time spent with practitioners?
- Do you think that internet pharmaceutical services are good for repeat prescriptions, and therefore represents a genuine service to the public?
- Do you think that these services should be more subject to control?
- What about 'natural substances' – would you prefer that these are less regulated, or do you think that some practitioner assistance should be sought?
- Do you resent e-mails that are unsolicited, that offer life enhancement?
- Why do you think that such services flourish?

References

1. Merriam-Webster, Merriam-Webster's Medical Dictionary. In *Merriam-Webster's Online Dictionary and Thesaurus*, Merriam-Webster: 2012.
2. WHO *The World Health Organisation Report: Working Together for Health*; World Health Organisation: Geneva, 2006.
3. Talbott Recovery Campus, Talbott Medication Guide. Talbott Pharmaceutical Company: 2008. http://www.talbottcampus.com (accessed 13 October 2012).
4. Yano, R.; Ohtsu, F.; Goto, N., Relationship between Physicochemical Properties of Medical Supplies and Serious Adverse Drug Reactions Listed in the Package Inserts. *Yakugaku Zasshi* **2017**.
5. Fox, E. R.; Sweet, B. V.; Jensen, V., Drug Shortages: A Complex Health Care Crisis. *Mayo Clinic Proceedings* **2014,** *89* (3), 361-373.
6. Kasciuskeviciute, S.; Gumbrevicius, G.; Vendzelyte, A.; Sciupokas, A.; Petrikonis, K.; Kadusevicius, E., Impact of the World Health Organization Pain Treatment Guidelines and the European Medicines Agency Safety Recommendations on Nonsteroidal Anti-Inflammatory Drug Use in Lithuania: An Observational Study. *Medicina (Kaunas)* **2018,** *54* (2).
7. Leenen, F. H. H.; Dumais, J.; McInnis, N. H.; Turton, P.; Stratychuk, L.; Nemeth, K.; Lum-Kwong, M. M.; Fodor, G., Results of the Ontario Survey on the Prevalence and Control of Hypertension. *Canadian Medical Association Journal* **2008,** *178* (11), 1441-9.
8. Alves, R. R.; Rosa, I. M. Biodiversity, traditional medicine and public health: where do they meet? *Journal of Ethnobiology and Ethnomedicine* [Online], 2007. (accessed 4th September 2007).
9. Murray, M. T.; Pizzorno, J. E., Nutritional Medicine. In *The Textbook of Natural Medicine*, 3rd ed.; Pizzorno, J. E.; Murray, M. T., Eds. Churchill Livingstone Elsevier: St Louis, 2006; Vol. 1.
10. Barber, R. M.; Fullman, N.; Sorensen, R. J. D.; Bollyky, T.; McKee, M.; Nolte, E.; al., e. Healthcare Access and Quality Index based on mortality from causes amenable to personal health care in 195 countries and territories, 1990-2015: a novel analysis from the Global Burden of Disease Study 2015 *The Lancet* [Online], 2017. http://dx.doi.org/10.1016/S0140-6736(17)30818-8 (accessed 27 May 2017).
11. Bradley, R. S., Philosophy of Natural Medicine. In *The Textbook of Natural Medicine*, 3rd ed.; Pizzorno, J. E.; Murray, M. T., Eds. Churchill Livingstone Elsevier: St Louis, 2006; Vol. 1.
12. Bayliss, E. A.; Steiner, J. F.; Fernald, D. H.; Crane, L. A.; Main, D. S., Descriptions of barriers to self-care by persons with comorbid chronic diseases. *Annals of Family Medicine* **2003,** (1), 15-21.
13. Barnes, J.; Anderson, L. A.; Phillipson, J. D., Herbal Interactions. *The Pharmaceutical Journal* **2003,** *270*, 118-121.
14. De Busk, R. M., Integrative Medicine and Phytotherapy. In *Krause's Food Nutrition and Diet Therapy*, 11th ed.; Mahan, L. K.; Escott-Stump, S., Eds. Elsevier: Philadelphia, 2004.

15. Sutherst, R. W. Global Change and Human Vulnerability to Vector-Borne Diseases *Clinical Microbiology Reviews* [Online], 2004, p. 136-173. (accessed 4th September 2007).

16. WHO *A Safer Future: Global Health Security in the 21st Century*; World Health Organisation: Geneva, 2007.

17. Cassini, A.; Högberg, L. D.; Plachouras, D.; Quattrocchi, A.; Hoxha, A.; Simonsen, G. S.; et al., Attributable deaths and disability-adjusted life-years caused by infections with antibiotic-resistant bacteria in the EU and the European Economic Area in 2015: a population-level modelling analysis. *The Lancet Infectious Diseases* **2018**.

18. Ahmad, N.; Javaid, A.; Sulaiman, S. A.; Ming, L. C.; Ahmad, I.; Khan, A. H., Resistance patterns, prevalence, and predictors of fluoroquinolones resistance in multidrug-resistant tuberculosis patients. *Brazilian Journal of Infectious Diseases* **2016,** *20* (1), 41-7.

19. Sussman, S.; Sussman, A. N. Considering the Definition of Addiction *International Journal of Environmental Research and Public Health* [Online], 2011, p. 4025-4038. www.mdpi.com/journal/ijerph (accessed 8 October 2012).

20. Sussman, S.; Lisha, N.; Griffiths, M., Prevalence of the Addictions: A Problem of the Majority or the Minority? *Evaluation of Health Profession* **2011,** *34* (1), 3-56.

21. Solinas, M.; Yasar, S.; Goldberg, S. R., Endocannabinoid system involvement in brain reward processes related to drug abuse. *Pharmacological research : the official journal of the Italian Pharmacological Society* **2007,** *56* (5), 393-405.

22. Wu, L.-T.; Schlenger, W. E.; Galvin, D. M., Concurrent Use of Methamphetamine, MDMA, LSD, Ketamine, GHB, and Flunitrazepam among American Youths. *Drug and alcohol Dependance* **2006,** *84* (1), 102-113.

23. Connor, T. J. Methylenedioxymethamphetamine (MDMA, Ecstacy): a stressor on the immune system *Immunology* [Online], 2004, p. 357-367. (accessed 31 May 2008).

24. Bellis, M. A.; Hughes, K. E.; Dillon, P.; Copeland, J.; Gates, P. Effects of backpacking holidays in Australia on alcohol, tobacco and drug use of UK residents *Biomed Central: Public Health* [Online], 2007. http://www.biomedcentral.com/1471-2458/7/1 (accessed 31st May 2008).

25. Barker, J. C.; Harris, N. G.; Dyer, J. E., Experiences of Gamma-Hydroxybutyrate (GHB) Ingestion: A Focus Group Study. *Journal of Psychoactive Drugs* **2007,** *39* (2), 115-129.

26. Ali, A.; Arif, A. W.; Bhan, C.; Kumar, D.; Malik, M. B.; Sayyed, Z.; Akhtar, K. H.; Ahmad, M. Q., Managing Chronic Pain in the Elderly: An Overview of the Recent Therapeutic Advancements. *Cureus* **2018,** *10* (9), e3293.

27. Arria, A. M.; Garnier-Dykstra, L. M.; Caldeira, K. M.; Vincent, K. B.; O'Grady, K. E. Prescription Analgesic Use Among Young Adults: Adherence to Physician Instructions and Diversion *Pain Medicine* [Online], 2011, p. 898-903. (accessed 8 October 2012).

28. Gardner-Nix, J., Principles of opioid use in chronic noncancer pain. *Canadian Medical Association Journal* **2003,** *169* (1), 38-43.

29. Simoni-Wastila, L.; Strickler, G., Risk Factors Associated with Problem Use of Prescription Drugs. *American Journal of Public Health* **2004,** *94* (2), 266-268.

30. *House of Lords Select Committee on Science and Technology - Sixth Report on Complementary and Alternative Medicine*; House of Lords: London, November 2000, 2000.

LEARNING SESSION SIX: MOVEMENT AND HEALTH

Introduction

We explore here the connection not only between exercise, movement and health but also between movement and self-expression. We look at both the curative aspects of movement as well as those that are preventative and how engaging in some form of exercise can be part of a good health insurance policy for the future. In addition to physical health, the mental and emotional aspects of movement are equally important. How you exercise, and the form of exercise that you prefer is a part of your personality and can be an expression of one's own goals and aspirations.

There are many ways in which one can engage with movement from traditional dancing to modern equipped gymnasiums. Team sports can be competitive and may be a way of providing the impetus for those who find it hard to motivate themselves, or it may simply be a way of getting together with friends. Gentler non-competitive group activities such as yoga are more suitable for those who would rather not raise the adrenalin levels. For some, a walk in the park and home gardening provide a way of giving oneself some mental space while engaging in health-enhancing movement. Some of the means of movement require membership of a club or gym; others do not. We look at the overall benefits of exercise before coming to our first learning together session, where we explore some of the options available to us.

It is possible for each of us to find something we enjoy doing with a little searching around, and in our second learning together session we look at the cheap and easy options, the benefits of groups and how to start an exercise group of one's own. Finally, we come to our discussion of the day, how much is enough and how much is too much, is more, better, or can exercise be overdone and become addictive, over competitive and stressful?

Ice-Breaker Quiz

Let us look at the benefits of exercise and see how well we are doing and whether there is a way to get more out of this:

A. Which of the following would you rate as being a benefit of exercise and movement?

Better sleep   Fresh air   Stress management   Weight control

Enjoyment   Social contact   Quality time with family

Cardiovascular fitness   Muscular strength   Better balance

Sunshine   Suppleness

Time to yourself   Decreasing boredom   Improving appetite

Making friends   Relaxation   Mood improvement

Winning sports competitions   Teambuilding

B. Decide on the five which are most important to you
C. Place your score of how well, on average, you are doing by each item on your list

Awesome! = 5   Sharp = 4   OK = 3   Poor = 2   Gross = 1

1. _____

2. _____

3. _____

4. _____

5. _____

Movement, Health and Self-Expression

Exercise is one of the cornerstones of both preventative and anti-ageing medicine and holds promise for the prevention of degenerative disease and delaying the ageing process [1]. It is economically and technologically more advantageous to keep the older generation healthy and active within the global community and to our great collective disadvantage to having an ageing society which becomes a burden [1]. Older bereaved persons who engage in regular physical activity as well as watching the quantity and quality of their dietary intake as well as getting a get a good night's sleep, are more likely to recover from their bereavement psychologically and emotionally and are less likely to suffer illness and physical degeneration as a result [2]. Exercise, in conjunction with diet, nutritional supplements and stress management is as important an issue for the health care profession and, in particular, for the prevention of degeneration as any other aspect of medicine [1]. The habits of exercise, however, begin when one is young and the longer these activities are kept up, the more beneficial they become, as one goes through life.

It is not only ageing and degenerative disorders that are of concern, however, as a particular group of disorders has arisen recently as a major threat to health, namely that of obesity, a major independent risk factor for cardiac disease [3]. More than half of US citizens are either overweight or obese [3]. To date, the causes of this epidemic alongside its sister disorder, metabolic syndrome, have been investigated by a number of scientific teams [4]. Although metabolic factors do play a role, the predominant causes are laid squarely at the foot of too high a consumption of high fat, high refined carbohydrate foods and too little exercise [4]. Regular exercise is a major factor in the prevention of cardiovascular disease and has also been implicated in the prevention of a number of cancers, including those of prostate, colon, breast and endometrial cancer [5]. Conversely, it is estimated that physical inactivity is responsible for approximately 250,000 premature deaths per year [5].

Despite the fact that the results of inactivity, as well as the benefits of regular exercise, have been well understood for a number of years, exercise interventions amongst high-risk populations have largely failed [5]. Research is now more focussed on why this has been the case and what the possible motivational aspects of exercise might be. Ways to both promote and sustain physical activity must be found to prevent disease and premature deaths in the future. Perhaps a broader view of exercise and the connection between movement and self-expression needs to be reviewed, to open the possibilities for sustained and regular movement and to enhance the pleasure of doing it.

The call for physical activity is neither new nor particularly a concept of Western civilisation, with its gyms and competitive sports activities. In Asia, the importance of exercise and its connection to health and longevity was recognised more than 4,000 years ago [6]. Approximately 2,500 years ago, the Greek civilisation also proclaimed the importance of physical activity [6] and the Olympic games are still with us today as a test of strength and endurance, speed and skill.

Exercise, however, can embrace just about any kind of physical movement and is not required to be strenuous, onerous or monotonous. Movement can be part of socialising and pleasure as well as a form of self-expression. The motivation to exercise is more easily and readily sustained, in fact, if the movement one is engaged in brings pleasure and enhances mood [5].

Brain-derived neurotrophic factor (BDNF) is a substance that promotes repair and enhancement of certain regions of the brain, spinal cord, vascular and central nervous systems [5]. Deficiencies in BDNF have been shown to increase one's chances of depression and nervous disorders; however, to some extent, the ability of the body to produce this is genetic [5]. Some people simply have more of it than others. This is not a case of despair for the 'have not's' of BDNF, this substance is enhanced by exercise in any form at all – hence the generation of the 'feel good factor' in exercise [5]. It is this factor that helps the body to set up a 'loop' between exercise, physical regeneration, feeling good and being motivated to continue to exercise. Breaking into this loop need not be difficult, expensive or out of the ordinary. Movement can be part and parcel of who you are, a reflection of your culture, and a way of engaging in social life, as well as maintaining a balanced perspective in a world which is becoming aesthetic and devoid of a tradition for many urban dwellers.

Dancing is a cross-cultural medium of expression that pervades every society and ethnic identity. The value of this for both health and self-expression cannot be underestimated. Regardless of age, dancing is something that most people can manage from the time they can walk, until well into advanced age [7]. Social dancing in older people has been found to improve balance, stride and stability when walking, thus reducing the potential for falls, a source of major injury in the elderly population [7]. Dancing enhances not only physical fitness but also social skills, thus improving mental well-being and cognitive ability throughout life [8].

To benefit socially and psychologically the best forms of dancing to take up are those that encourage and develop cooperation, such as formation dancing (circle dancing, square dancing, line dancing). Playford English country dancing and American square dancing are taken at a walking pace and are good for older persons, and those with limited mobility and energy problems. They require, however, increasingly complex movements which develop coordination and neurological function [8]. Ballroom and Latin American dancing require an equally skilled partner but increase cardiovascular fitness, the fluidity of movement, balance and coordination [8].

Dog walking is often overlooked as an exercise medium, but research has found that there are considerable benefits, not only physically but socially and psychologically [9]. A pet is a part of one's household or family and in some measure an extension of the family values. Pets require care and involve a measure of responsibility, in turn, however, they give back affection, protection and companionship, and increase social contact [9].

Quick Quiz

Below is a random assortment of types of exercise which fall into two groups, those that have a traditional cultural basis and a distinctive ethnic origin and those that are more modern, and possibly based on medical research. See if you can distinguish between the two.

Yoga   Resistance weight training   English country dancing

Circuit training   Running   Lawn Croquet

Tai chi   Pilates   Circle dancing   Gymnastics

Step dancing   Spinning

Traditional Exercise

1. _____

2. _____

3. _____

4. _____

5. _____

6. _____

Modern Exercise

1. _____

2. _____

3. _____

4. _____

5. _____

6. _____

Ways-to-go: Different Types of Movement and Benefits

There are five components of physical fitness, all of which have specific benefits to specific physical systems in our bodies [10]. These are:

- Cardiovascular endurance
- Muscular strength
- Muscular endurance
- Flexibility
- Body composition (the ratio of fat to lean tissue and bone strength)

On the whole, exercise falls into two broad categories, that of aerobic exercise, i.e. that which uses up oxygen and for the main conditions the cardiovascular system, and non-aerobic exercise which tones and strengthens muscle tissue [10].

Cardiovascular endurance

Exercises which build up cardiovascular endurance include those of:

- Walking, jogging or running
- Dance – especially rhythmic, aerobic, ballroom and Latin American as well as line dancing and other traditional forms of dancing including Scottish and Irish traditional dancing
- Swimming

Any form of aerobic exercise is beneficial not only to the cardiovascular system but also to the problem of disordered breathing as well. Research has demonstrated that snoring, a problem of sleep-disordered breathing, is greatly improved by regular aerobic exercise even at a relatively low-intensity level [11]. This is a safe activity for children as well as adults and could, in fact, deal with several obesity-related problems at once, those of disordered breathing and snoring as well as the central problem of obesity [11].

Dance or movement therapy, which usually employs a combination of structured and unstructured movements, can be an important complement to other forms of therapy that are commonly used to alleviate long-lasting and chronic pain [12]. Dance therapy has also been shown to help people overcome health problems that result in physical limitations and disability as well as psychological distress, and to foster their self-esteem or self-concept [12]. Dance therapy can not only induce relaxation and improve muscle tone; it can also increase flexibility and joint range of motion [12]. Among those who participate in dance therapy, it has been observed that the process of movement based on a specific theme, often elicits memories that can be discussed in a group. This outcome potentially increases their opportunities for social contact, support, and self-expression, deemed to promote health status [12]. It has also been observed that dance-based aerobic exercises can improve the balance capacity, as well as the walking and agility profile of the participant [12]. Moreover, performed individually or in a group, dance-based therapy may be extremely helpful for encouraging and improving the mobility and functional capacity of people with arthritis, especially older adults, who cannot participate in vigorous or stressful aerobic exercises [12].

Walking is probably the safest, cheapest and easiest form of exercise that can be done at home on an unsupervised basis even for those with little physical fitness at the onset. Research has shown that even for individuals with a high risk of cardiovascular disease, or who have already had a major cardiac event, a gradated walking programme can be initiated [13]. Any medical problem that ensues is not likely to be as a result of walking but, to date, has been found to be due to other health-related factors [13]. In the treatment of type 2 diabetes walking as a form of regular exercise compared favourably to an individually structured exercise programme. The medical benefits were not different, but long term adherence was greater with the group walking [14].

All the above exercises, in addition to building cardiovascular endurance, will also strengthen muscles, correct body composition and build and strengthen the bone structure, thus having multiple benefits to those who participate. Swimming is perhaps the exception in that this and other exercises performed in water are relatively non-weight bearing, that is they do not strengthen or build bone as they do not exert much stress on the bone structure. This, however, can be of benefit to persons recovering from bone injuries, the morbidly obese who cannot initially tolerate stress on the bone structure and those who have bone-related pathologies such as Paget's disease or osteoarthritis.

Muscular strength, endurance and flexibility

Resistance exercises such as working with light to medium weights or those which use the body's own weight as resistance such as sit-ups and push-ups increase the strength, tone and endurance of the skeletal-muscular system. Most of these exercises will also increase bone density and enhance bone strength [10]. Flexibility is the ability to move a muscle through its full range of motion and involves the interrelationship of muscles, tendons and joints conditioning this whole integrated system. Two special kinds of exercise which do not require the use of equipment are worth mentioning here. Yoga and Tai Chi are well-tried forms of movement that not only enhance muscle strength but also increase the condition of internal organs, as well as flexibility and balance. Research has also shown that these forms of exercise are in addition, good alleviators of stress.

Tai Chi is a form of traditional Chinese exercise that purports to improve health by changes in mental focus, breathing, coordination and relaxation. The goal of Tai Chi is to 'rebalance' the body's own healing capacity. As opposed to many forms of Western-style exercise, the remarkable benefits of Tai Chi are achieved by performing slow-speed, gentle, fluid, self-paced continuous graceful circular and non-impact movements of all body parts. Its movements, which incorporate deep breathing, while maintaining an upright posture are designed to soothe rather than stress, and very important in the context of arthritis, place no undue strain on muscles, joints, and connective tissues [12]. Tai Chi has been practised in China for hundreds of years and is now widely practised throughout the world [15]. Studies have shown that Tai Chi can help to improve balance and prevent falls in the elderly improve musculoskeletal conditions lower hypertension, enhance cardiovascular and respiratory function improve mental health and enhance endocrine and immune functioning [15].

As an intervention for headache, and arthritis, Tai Chi offers several benefits over conventional treatment [12]. Virtually all pharmaceutical-based interventions include some risk to the patient of side-effects or complications, particularly over a long-term course of use. Of the most widely utilized drugs for tension-type headaches (TTH), acetaminophen (the active ingredient in Tylenol) can cause liver toxicity, and non-steroidal anti-inflammatory drugs (NSAIDs) such as ibuprofen and aspirin can cause gastrointestinal symptoms and bleeding. To the extent that treatment can be refocused to exercise-based therapies, this will provide significant benefit to the patient [15].

Arthritis, in its various forms, as well as headaches, are the most common problems for which pain and NSAIDs are used on a long-term basis. According to the US National Headache Foundation, more than 45 million Americans suffer from chronic headaches, with losses of $50 billion a year to absenteeism and medical expenses and an excess of $4 billion spent on over-the-counter medications. The statistics may not be very different in other parts of the developed world. Tension-type headaches (TTH), which represent approximately 78% of all headaches, occur either in single episodes or chronically, and are often the result of temporary stress, anxiety, fatigue or anger [15].

Yoga is another ancient movement therapy of eastern (mainly Indian) origin that is also a slow movement and posture holding exercise similar to Tai Chi, which is rapidly gaining popularity in the West. Studies have found that yoga interventions have been successful in the reduction of body weight, blood pressure, cholesterol and blood glucose [16,17]. In addition, the overall quality of life amongst older yoga participants has also been found to improve significantly [17].

Learning Together

Activity 6.1: Allow approximately 15 minutes for this exercise.

There are sixteen forms of movement that can be found in this puzzle. For those who have not done a word search before, the letters of the words may run across, down or diagonally and may be spelt forwards or backwards. See if you can find them all. If you can, you will find that there are nine letters that do not form a part of any word – these spell the result of what you will get with good lifestyle management.

WORDSEARCH

Y	C	Y	C	L	I	N	G	N
G	O	L	F	S	W	I	M	O
N	W	G	W	P	W	O	R	T
I	E	T	A	I	C	H	I	N
C	J	E	L	L	R	U	N	I
N	O	N	K	A	E	S	I	M
A	G	N	I	T	A	K	S	D
D	L	I	N	E	G	I	N	A
B	L	S	G	S	L	W	O	B

You may now like to take five minutes to discuss this exercise.

Motivation and Movement: Finding Something You Like

Psychologists have long been interested in the question of motivation, and what may or may not motivate someone to do anything. Sociologists have looked instead at structures in society and which structures are encouraging and which are not [18]. Whichever way the question of motivation is viewed, it is unarguably a major factor in health and well-being as it is the prime driver behind both changes in respect of lifestyle and long-term maintenance of habits that eventually become ingrained lifestyle choices. It has been found that personality is a strong indicator of who will and will not engage in exercise. People who are positive, outgoing and sociable are more likely to engage in an exercise programme [19]. Those who are conscientious and self-disciplined are likely to maintain an exercise programme. In addition, knowledge of the benefits of health are also motivational as is self-sufficiency and the ability to make choices [20]. Self-centred people, who are negative in their outlook and those who engage in self-reproach are less likely to begin an exercise programme and if they do so are less likely to maintain it [19].

The lack of motivation is probably the one main barrier to exercise for most people. This might be due to external factors such as cost, availability of facilities or equipment, physiological factors such as pain, lack of endurance or insufficient energy or safety factors such as walking alone. There are two components to motivation; one is removing the barriers or finding some form of movement that fits with the resources at one's disposal. The other is an understanding of oneself and what is or is not psychologically suited to one's own personality, goals and desires for how to use free time. Motivation is an 'inside job', making it difficult to promote an exercise programme of any kind.

Health benefits of walking have been well-researched, but it has been found that barriers to walking include those of appearance (it looks naff!) footwear (I cannot wear walking boots) and situations (it gets dark early, or the area is unsafe or polluted) [21]. Some fears may be well-founded as in the US, both walking and cycling in large busy cities are both more dangerous than travelling by car [22]. It is possible, however, to achieve safe walking and cycling reducing accidents and fatalities on a national level as has been done in both The Netherlands and Germany by the implementation of local and national road safety policies that favour cyclists and pedestrians over vehicles [22]. Some people will make an excuse out of anything; however, it has been found that personality plays as large a role in exercise as does environment [19]. The intention to walk is facilitated and strengthened by an environment conducive to walking [19].

Interactive video games are a popular alternative to physical exercise for young people today. Research has demonstrated that this could be an answer to inactivity in children who are not as yet overweight but not particularly active as well as those who are obese or are heading towards obesity [23]. Interactive video dance games which match the level of interaction and play to increasing skill prove a 'cool' and highly successful way of sustaining motivation for youngsters, otherwise glued to 'the box' and less inclined to exercise [23].

Exercising in groups provides additional motivation over exercising alone [24], as will be discussed further on. Planning is a reinforcing factor of the initial intention to exercise, for when the activity has been planned, then some investment of time, and perhaps money, clothing and equipment has been made, which the individual will be reluctant to waste [19]. Building social contacts and social capital is important as both an antecedent to change and to improve quality of life as well as an outcome of it. In this wise, bonding together one's social life with an exercise programme can create a vicious circle that gives the best outcome of both socialising and exercise. Motivation in this case then becomes part and parcel of both the initiative to continue and the outcome of participation [18].

Quick Quiz

Can you decide on the benefits of the following types of exercise? Match the type of exercise in the left-hand column with the benefits in the right-hand column by linking them with a coloured pencil line:

Walking

Cycling
                               Cardiovascular fitness

Tai chi
                               Improving muscle tone

Swimming
                               Improving balance

Yoga
                               Building muscular strength

Pilates
                               Improving breathing

Basketball
                               Improving concentration

Line dancing
                               Decreasing mental stress

Resistance training
                               Increasing endurance

Horse riding
                               Decreasing body fat

Rock climbing
                               Contouring body shape

Aerobic dancing
                               Improving reaction time

Ice skating
                               Team building

Cheap and Easy Movement

Some forms of exercise require certain types of clothing or membership of a gym or club, while others require some organisation, cooperation and team building. There are some forms of exercise, however, for which one needs virtually no planning and no outlay. The most obvious of these is walking, which, despite its lowly origins and minimal outlay is physiologically the best exercise one can get as far as cardiovascular fitness is concerned. With the addition of a couple of handheld weights, one can also build in a muscle toning regime to the walk. Walking is the best form of exercise if one is overweight, unused to exercise, or has arthritis, previous injuries, or if one is recovering from illness. Walking has increased only slightly over the last 40 years [25] and evidence suggests that people most often walk because they have to rather than for pleasure [19]. However, walking is greatly underrated, and there are additional positive effects when walking in green spaces or even along a quiet tree-lined street, that goes well beyond that of just exercise. Walking in such environments has been shown to reduce stress, decrease aggression and even lower crime rates [19]!

In addition, there are other forms of exercise that are just as beneficial for similar reasons, they are conducted outdoors, amongst greener environments, promote mental and emotional relaxation, while being a good form of movement for health. In particular, gardening has such benefits [19] as it is not only inexpensive but can be put to good economic use in growing food, even if it is only the more expensive kitchen herbs that one would otherwise buy. Cycling is also inexpensive and can save some money on transport. It can both be used as a means of getting to and from school or work, and for other regular short trips, as a hobby, done alone, or in a group. It equally has the benefit of cardiovascular exercise and getting outdoors into the fresh air, sunshine and green spaces [26]. All three of these forms of movement are, in addition, more likely to be sustained over a longer period of time than expensive high-tech indoor pursuits that require structured time, money and supervision [26].

The Benefits of Groups

Exercising in a group is generally more motivational as the group becomes cohesive, and the participant identifies with the group. Studies have found that, for older people, especially those living alone, the exercise group becomes their 'exercise family' [24]. Apart from the physical benefits gained from the exercise, significant emotional and psychological benefits are also gained when exercising in a group [24]. The maintenance of cognitive abilities in older people is significant, and there is an increased ability to function socially across the board [24]. Places of religion and cultural organisations who organise such exercise groups provide an added dimension to the exercise groups, as participants will have more than the motivation to exercise in common and will often make lasting friendships in the group which provide an additional motivating factor [24].

Exercising with friends and family are also strongly motivational and those who engage in exercising with friends, or as a family, have been found to be more likely to continue the exercise programme over a longer period of time [20]. For outdoor pursuits, there is, in addition, a safety factor that might make the difference between exercising or not exercising, especially when walking or cycling in cities [26] or hiking over a distance. In addition, walking in a familiar environment where one is likely to meet people one knows, thereby enhancing the social contact element of exercise, increases the frequency of walking, and is a likely factor in sustaining exercise [26].

Social cohesion and social capital per se are health-enhancing behaviours, and research has found that group participation and group encouragement is a health-promoting factor in life. The overall viewpoint holds that the more we stick together at just about anything, the more likely we are to keep up a level of health beyond that of conducting our lives in a more isolated or individualistic manner [27,28].

Learning Together

Activity 6.2: Take approximately 15 minutes for this exercise

We now come to a little creative decision making, for which we need to get into groups that, if possible, encompass more than one culture or point of view. Together in these groups, we are going to find a requirement in one culture, and away of fulfilling that requirement, that has a physical benefit, that comes from another culture.

The criteria are:
1. The requirement must be genuine and basic
2. The physical activity that meets it should be inexpensive, low-tech and done in a group

To follow is an example:
Requirement: Children need to be able to walk safely to school as the bus is becoming too expensive (and the world's fuel use must be curtailed). A typical Southern African problem!

Met by: A group of pensioners, one at the front, one at the rear and two in the middle create a walking bus, escorting the children to and from\school. A typical American solution to beat hypertension and obesity!

Do not limit yourselves and do not think about how usual or unusual your answers might be as even the wackiest ideas might spark a seed of hope in the great arena of problem-solving!

You may now like to take five minutes to discuss these answers.

Group Discussion

HOW MUCH IS ENOUGH AND HOW MUCH IS JUST A STEP (OR MANY) TOO FAR?

Exercise is good for you; it enhances health and well-being, can be a mean of releasing stress, can relax as well as invigorate and, in some respects, can provide a means of cultural and / or self-expression. Gym consortiums have become big business, and (to an extent) memberships have become an ultra-modern 'must have'. One can become addicted to the adrenalin rush of frequent excessive exercise and, the cost of a pair of designer trainers is more than a month's wages in the financial lower third of the world's countries. Taking these two facts into consideration, we need to ask ourselves how much should one be doing and how much should this 'doing' cost us?

References

1. Grossman T. Latest advances in anti-ageing medicine. Keio Journal of Medicine. 2005;54(2):85-94.

2. Chen JH, Gill TM, Prigerson HG. Health Behaviours Associated with Better Quality of Life for Older Bereaved Persons. Journal of Palliative Medicine. 2005;8(1):96-106.

3. Kokkinos P, Moutsatsos G. Obesity and Cardiovascular Disease. Journal of Cardiopulmonary Rehabilitation. 2004;24:197-204.

4. Bloomgarden ZT. Obesity, Hypertension, and Insulin Resistance. Diabetes Care. 2002;25(11):2088-99.

5. Bryan A, Hutchison KE, Seals DR, Allen DL. A Transdisciplinary Model Integrating Genetic, Physiological and Psychological Correlates of Voluntary Exercise. Health Psychology. 2007;26(1):30-9.

6. Paffenbarger RS, Olsen E. LifeFit. Champaigne, Illinois, USA: Human Kinetics Books; 1996.

7. Verghese J. Cognitive and Mobility Profile of Older Social Dancers. Journal of the American Geriatric Society. 2006;54(8):1241-4.

8. Bremer Z. Dance as a form of exercise. British Journal of General Practice. 2007:166.

9. Cutt HE, Knuiman MW, Giles-Corti B. Does getting a dog increase recreational walking? Biomed Central International Journal of Behavioural Nutrition and Physical Activity. Volume 5, 2008.

10. Lutack B, Bongiorno PB. The Exercise Prescription. In: Pizzorno JE, Murray MT (eds). Textbook of Natural Medicine. 3rd ed. Volume 1. St Louis: Churchill Livingstone Elsevier, 2006.

11. Davis CL, Tkacz J, Gregoski M, Boyle CA, Loverekovic G. Aerobic Exercise and Snoring in Overweight Children: A Randomised Controlled Trial. Obesity 2006;14(11):1985-91.

12. Marks R. Dance-based exercise and Tai Chi and their benefits for people with arthritis: a review. Health Education. 2005;105(5):374-91.

13. Goodrich DE, Larkin AR, Lowery JC, Holleman RG, Richardson CR. Adverse events among high-risk participants in a home based walking study: a descriptive study. Biomed Central International Journal of Behavioural Nutrition and Physical Activity. Volume 4, 2007.

14. Praet SFE, van-Rooij ESJ, Wijtvliet A, et al. Brisk walking compared with an individualised medical fitness programme for patients with type 2 diabetes: a randomised controlled trial. Diabetologia. Volume 51, 2008:736-46.

15. Abbott RB, Hui K-K, Hays RD, Li M-D, Pan T. A Randomized Controlled Trial of Tai Chi for Tension Headaches. Complementary and Alternative Medicine. Volume 4, 2007:107-13.

16. Yang K. A Review of Yoga Programs for Four Leading Risk Factors of Chronic Diseases. Complementary and Alternative Medicine. Volume 4, 2007:487-91.

17. Oken BS, Zajdel D, Kishiyama S, et al. Randomised Controlled Six-Month Trial of Yoga in Healthy Seniors: Effects on Cognition and Quality of Life. Alternative Therapies Health and Medicine. 2006;12(1):40-7.

18. Kahana E, Kahana B, Zhang J. Motivational Antecedents of Preventative Proactivity in Late LifeL Linking Future Orientation and Exercise. Motivation and Emotion. 2005;29(4):438=59.

19. Rhodes RE, Courneya KS, Blanchard CM, Plotnikoff RC. Prediction of leisure-time walking: an integration of social cognitive, perceived environmental and personality factors. Biomed Central International Journal of Behavioural Nutrition and Physical Activity. Volume 4, 2007.

20. Boutelle KN, Jeffery RW, French SA. Predictors of vigorous exercise adoption and maintenance over four years in a community sample. International Journal of Behavioural Nutrition and Physical Activity. Volume 1, 2004.

21. Dunton GF, Schneider M. Perceived Barriers to Walking for Physical Activity. Preventing Chronic Disease. Volume 3, 2006.

22. Pucher J, Dijkstra L. Promoting Safe Walking and Cycling to Improve Public Health: Lessons from The Netherlands and Germany. American Journal of Public Health. 2003;93(9):1509-16.

23. Epstein LH, Beecher MD, Graf JL, Roemmich JN. Choice of Interactive Dance and Bicycle Games in Overweight and Nonoverweight Youth. Annals of Behavioural Medicine. 2007;33(2):124-31.

24. Chiang K-C, Seman L, Belza B, Tsai JH-C. "It Is Our Exercise Family": Experiences of Ethnic Older Adults in a Group-Based Exercise Programme. Preventing Chronic Disease. Volume 5, 2008.

25. Tudor-Locke C, van-der-Ploeg HP, Bowles HR, et al. Walking behaviours from the 1965-2003 American Heritage Time Use Study (AHTUS). International Journal of Behavioural Nutrition and Physical Activity. Volume 4, 2007.

26. Shephard RJ. What is the optimal type of physical activity to enhance health? British Journal of Sports Medicine. 1997;31:277-84.

27. Oishi S, Koo M. Culture, Interpersonal Perceptions and Happiness in Social Interactions. Personal and Social Psychology Bulletins. 2008;34(3):307-20.

28. Peterson J, Atwood JR, Yates B. Key Elements for Church-Based Health Promotion Programs: Outcome-Based Literature Review. Public Health Nursing. 2002;19(6):401-11.

LEARNING SESSION SEVEN: THE ELEMENTS OF LIFE

Introduction

Here we look at the elements we need to survive, what they are, and why they are essential and, most importantly, what they have to do with a programme on lifestyle management! Water, air and sunlight are essential to all growth, whether that of plants, animals or human beings. We discover how and why these are important to human life. We look at the issue of adequate hydration, the quality of our air and the appropriate amount of sunlight necessary to health, and how to gain the maximum benefit with the minimum damage.

Water is a bit controversial these days, it not only comes out of the tap (for most of us that is) but also in bottles of varying types and qualities which we might boil, filter, or add substances to. We look at our body's needs for water, the signs and symptoms of dehydration, and how to avoid this problem. We also look at obtaining the best quality water that we can, given our circumstances, and the best ways to consume fluids. In our first learning session, we learn how to calculate our individual fluid requirements.

We then go on to air, clean air and good quality air as well as the correct way to breathe. We look at what happens when we are only slightly short of oxygen and how to get a good supply under less than ideal circumstances. Finally, we look at sunlight which we need, not only as a source of vitamin D but also to build an essential neurotransmitter, serotonin. We look at what happens when we have too little as well as too much, and how to maintain a sensible balance. In our second group learning activity, we engage in some interesting and fun ideas for improving both the condition of our air and our nutrition. We then move on to our discussion for this session – seeing the trees for more than the woods. Although we need land for agriculture, can we find a balance – what is in a tree for us?

Ice-Breaker Quiz

So how much do you know about your essential needs for water, air and sunshine before we begin? Without looking any further, let's see how you do in the following multiple-choice questions:

1. The human body is comprised mainly of

    A. Stored Fat
    B. Bone
    C. Muscular tissues
Answer: _____
    D. Water

2. The first sign of dehydration is

    A. Thirst
    B. Fatigue
    C. Headache
Answer: _____
    D. Bad breath

3. The correct amount of time one should be exposed to the sun without sun cream is

    A. Never
    B. 10 minutes
    C. 15 minutes
Answer: _____
    D. 30 minutes

4. Shallow breathing is:

    A. A sign of Asthma
    B. A symptom of a panic attack
    C. The way most people breathe
    D. The correct way of breathing
Answer: _____

5. Sun exposure is best avoided:

    A. Between 10.00 and 15.00
    B. After Noon
    C. Before noon
    D. During the three summer months of the year
Answer: _____

Water and Hydration

Water is the largest single component of the body, and the volume, distribution and composition of the body fluids have profound effects on the function of the individual cells, tissues organs, and the metabolic balance of the body. The cells of the muscles and viscera have the highest water content in the body, whereas the calcified tissues of bones and teeth have the least. Athletes, and those with a relatively high proportion of lean body mass, have a higher body water content than those who are less active and, as one ages, and the lean tissue mass depletes, the water content of the body also diminishes [1]. On average, a healthy man of average weight and fitness will have a total body water content of 60% and a healthy average woman a total body water content of 55% [2].

Of the total body water content, 2/3 will be intracellular fluid, that is the fluid inside the cells, and 1/3 extracellular fluid, that is the fluid outside of the cells. Much of this (80%) is the fluid surrounding the cells, commonly termed 'interstitial fluid' and 20% is plasma (the liquid portion of the blood) [2]. This is shown better in the chart below.

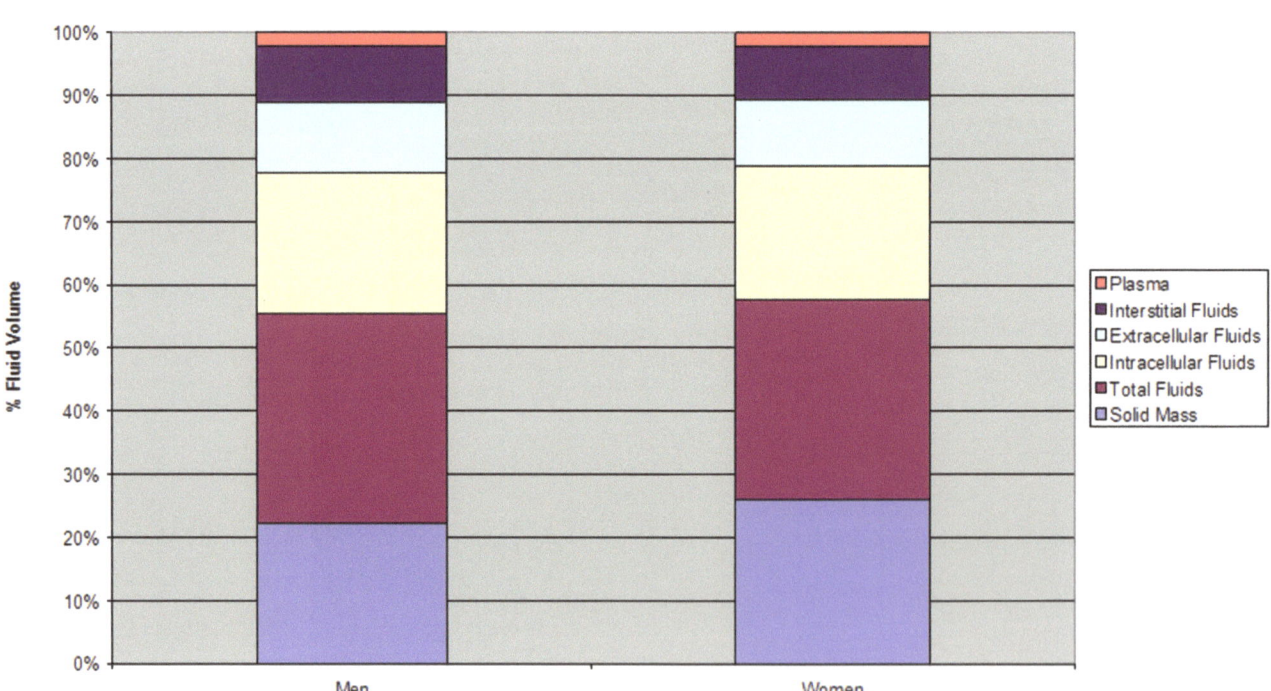

Source: author's own construction

Water is the universal solvent and is vital for all the body's enzymatic and metabolic functions. The body has no ability to store water, and the water lost each day needs to be replenished. Water comes from only one of three sources: foods, fluid intake and water of metabolism, which is the water yielded from the chemical conversion of food to energy. The water of metabolism accounts for between 200 ml and 300 ml of water per day, depending on the amount of food eaten and, the efficiency of its conversion. The remainder needs to be taken in via the food and beverage content of the diet [1].

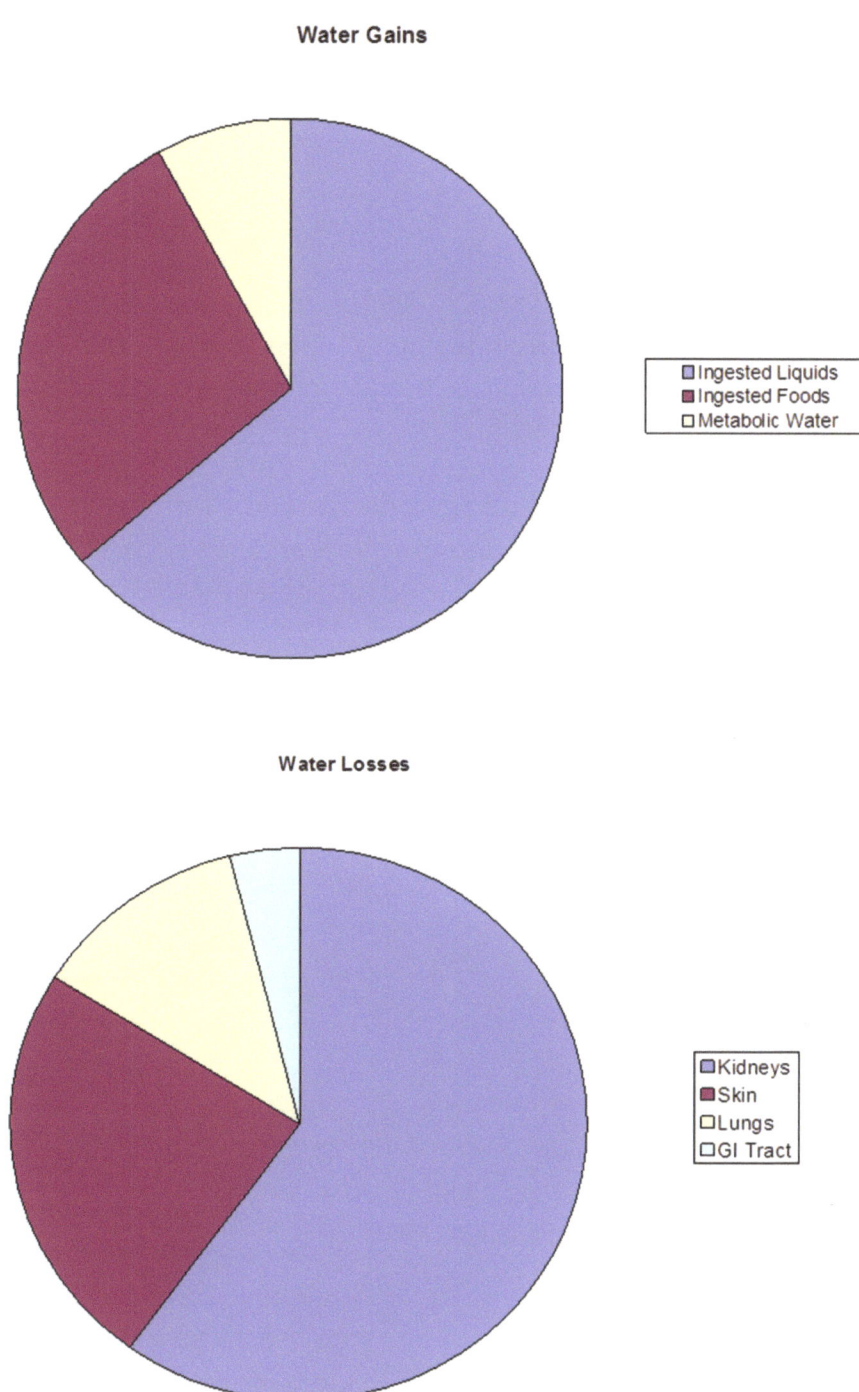

Water Gains

Ingested Liquids
Ingested Foods
Metabolic Water

Water Losses

Kidneys
Skin
Lungs
GI Tract

Source: author's own construction

Total water gains need to meet the total water losses of approximately 2,500 ml per day. Approximately 1,600 ml is lost from kidneys and 100 ml in the faeces, another 600 ml is lost from skin and 300 ml from lungs [2].

When the required amount of water taken in by ingestion and the water of metabolism equals the water lost, then the body is said to be in *fluid balance*. Much can go wrong with this balance and keeping the balance constant requires that the water of metabolism is generated via the generation of energy and that enough fluid is taken in as well as the correct foods [2]. When a diet is rich in fresh fruits, vegetables, cooked grains, pulses and fresh nuts which hold water, then less will have to be drunk. A fat rich and / or protein-rich diet, however, which contains few fruits and vegetables will not only yield less in fluids but may require more fluids to be digested, necessitating a greater fluid intake.

Dehydration occurs when water loss is greater than water intake, meaning that there is a decrease in the volume of water and an increase in osmolarity (the ability of the fluids to pass across the cell membranes) of the body. Water losses result first in fatigue, followed by thirst generated by a feedback mechanism resulting from the increase in osmolarity. The body needs only to lose 2% of its mass due to fluid loss for mild dehydration to occur, and the symptoms of dehydration to be experienced [2].

Children and infants are at risk from mild dehydration with mild acute bouts of non-specific diarrhoea. The best treatment involves giving clear fluids such as cooled herbal teas (Rooibos / red bush tea contains minerals and antioxidants) and diluted clear apple juice are good choices. Current recommendations are that milk and dairy products should be stopped for at least 24 hours and the clear fluids given followed by the BRAT diet (bananas, rice cereal, applesauce and toast) and a probiotic [3]. Although the requirement for fluids is slightly less as one ages, there is a natural tendency for the sensation of thirst to diminish, making older persons more vulnerable to dehydration.

% of body weight lost through water losses	Symptoms of dehydration:
<1%	Fatigue
2	Thirst, vague discomfort and loss of appetite
3	Decreasing blood volume and impaired physical performance
4	Increased effort for physical work, nausea
5	Difficulty in concentrating
6	Failure to regulate body temperature
8	Dizziness, laboured breathing on exertion and increased weakness
10	Muscle spasms, delirium and wakefulness
11	Circulatory collapse and kidney failure

Chronic mild dehydration that is not necessarily clinically detectable, but is due to long term slightly inadequate fluid intake, is associated with constipation, an increased risk of kidney stones, decreased salivation and an increased risk of certain cancers as well as childhood obesity [1]. Increased fluid intake is also necessary with increased ambient temperature, sunbathing, exposure, exercise and increased perspiration due to strenuous exercise. Infection, illness, fever and stress will also increase the body's requirement for fluids as will fasting, decreased appetite and long periods spent in dry air-conditioned surroundings [1].

Dehydration due to insufficient water intake (as opposed to increased water losses) is more common in older people, often misdiagnosed or under-diagnosed and is associated with increased illness, adverse health outcomes, longer hospital stays and increased risk of death [4]. Dehydrated older people have a 40% risk of dying within the next 8 years, compared with those who are well-hydrated [4]. In older people, dehydration can develop over a long period of time and may be due to long-term chronically insufficient fluid intake [4].

Water balance, for practical purposes, is maintained by that which is ingested. Provided that five portions of fruits and vegetables are taken in, alongside other fresh foods which contain enough fluid for their own digestion, 1600 ml of water is needed as drinking water [2]. This applies to those of average weight, height and build and living in a temperate climate; however, there is a more exact way of calculating fluid needs [1], which we will go through in our 'group learning activity'. Water can be obtained in several ways, some of which are a better source of fluids than others. In order of choice these are [1]:

Pure water (with no change in taste, smell or colour)
Rooibos (red bush) tea
Fruit or herbal infusions
Clear diluted apple juice
Low sodium clear vegetable broth
Diluted clear fruit juices
Decaffeinated black tea
Freshly squeezed juices
Soda water
Light, thin soups

Milk and caffeinated drinks do not count towards the overall fluid intake for re-hydration purposes. Caffeinated drinks may exacerbate dehydration, as do alcoholic drinks [1]. Drinking water sources may need to be monitored, as research shows that both tap water and bottled waters contain varying amounts of minerals, especially calcium, magnesium and sodium. Magnesium and calcium, present in hard water, has been shown to decrease cardiac heart disease; however, soft water is high in sodium content and over time can increase the risk for this disease. Bottled water, if drunk on a continuous basis, may need compensating for in the rest of the food and fluid intake, especially if the sodium content is high [5]. Although filtering water for domestic use takes out some of the minerals, the chlorine used to decontaminate recycled water also leaves water exposed to further bacterial contamination [5]. This needs to be refrigerated and drunk within a few hours of filtering [5].

Learning Together

Activity 7.1: Allow 15 minutes for this activity

Hopefully, one member of each learning group will volunteer for this exercise, or choose someone between you, to calculate their fluid requirements. Now follow the steps below:

1. Take your volunteer's approximate weight in Kg
2. For the first ten Kg allow   1,000 ml
3. For the second 10 Kg allow   500 ml
4. For persons under 50 years allow 20 ml per Kg for the rest of the weight in Kg   ?
5. For persons older than 50 years allow 15 ml per Kg for the rest of the weight in Kg   ?

    <u>Sub Total</u>   _____

6. If the person is consuming three meals and two snacks per day (and therefore, taking in an average 2,500 Cal per day) deduct 200 ml
7. For each approximate 500 Cal over this, deduct another 50 ml

    <u>Sub Total</u>   _____

8. For each approximate 500 Cal under the average, add back to the subtotal above, 50 ml

EVERYONE
9. For each portion of fruit and vegetables consumed deduct 50 ml

TOTAL REQUIREMENTS   _____

Air and the Oxygen We Need

Although we traditionally think of respiration as something we do with our lungs, in fact, it is something we do with our cells. Respiration is the process of gas exchange in our bodies, and it has three basic steps [6]:

1. Pulmonary ventilation, or breathing, is the inflow and outflow of air between the atmosphere and the alveoli (small sponge-like tissues) of the lungs.
2. External respiration is the exchange of gases (oxygen and carbon dioxide) between the alveoli and the red blood cells.
3. Internal respiration is the exchange of gases between the red blood cells in the capillaries and the tissue cells of the organs of the body. Without this oxygen, the individual cells cannot produce energy or carry out any other metabolic chemical reaction.

To a large extent, all of this goes on without our conscious knowledge or control; however, the whole process begins with the pulmonary ventilation – breathing, which has two stages to it, that of inspiration (inhalation or breathing in) and expiration (exhalation or breathing out). Just before inspiration, the air pressure inside the lungs is equal to the pressure of the air outside. For air to flow in, the pressure inside needs to drop which is accomplished by the diaphragm (muscle at the base of the chest cavity) moving down to expand lung volume, allowing air to flow in. The oxygen then moves across the alveoli into the blood and cells, and the carbon dioxide is carried back to the lungs, through the alveoli and expired (breathed out). This is accomplished by the diaphragm moving up, contracting the lung capacity, creating higher pressure inside than outside and the air flows out [6].

There are two preconditions to all this happening with ease and for the body to obtain the right amount of oxygen for its needs. The first is that breathing is unobstructed, normal and without undue strain. The second is that the air we take in is clean, of good quality and has adequate oxygen content. The term for normal quiet breathing is *eupnoea* and which usually consists of a pattern of both shallow and deep breathing. Shallow breathing is known as **costal breathing** and consists of an upward and outward movement of the chest filling only the top ¼ to ½ of the lungs. A pattern of deep abdominal breathing where the diaphragm pulls down to its fullest extent, expanding the abdomen and filling the lungs completely is known as **diaphragmatic breathing** [6].

Bad breathing habits can be developed just as bad eating habits can be developed over time. Hyperventilation syndrome is a collection of problems caused by breathing pattern disorders. Some of these are due to an organic functional problem that requires medical diagnosis and correction; however, often acute hyperventilation can be due to nervous over-reaction to a stressful event, bronchial spasm, or an acute hypoglycaemic (low blood glucose) attack. A short-term problem can become a chronic long-term problem if not recognised and dealt with sufficiently. The good news is, however, that good breathing habits can be cultivated with correct breathing exercises, and a chronic shallow breather can learn to breathe deeply and evenly [6]. Physical therapy rehabilitation of breathing is summarised in the acronym [7]:

B	**B**reathing retraining
E	**E**steem / self-image
T	**T**otal body relaxation
T	**T**alk / breath control
E	**E**xercise prescription
R	**R**est / sleep

Although there is virtually no more debate about whether or not our world has become polluted, there is a considerable amount of debate as to whether or not the pollution has reached high enough levels to cause adverse effects [8]. Chronic obstructive pulmonary disease (COPD) is not an organic or functional disease due to an internal fault, or invasion by bacteria or viruses; it is solely because of breathing in noxious fumes and chemicals, the main cause of which is smoking. Asthma too is on the increase and is aggravated by poor air quality and stressful life situations [9-11].

In the last decade, the burden of disease in developing countries due to the use of biomass fuels (predominantly wood but also coal and charcoal) has been found to be significant. In India alone, approximately 400,000 – 550,000 premature deaths might be attributed to the damage done by the consistent use of biomass fuels. Women at home with children are predominantly at risk. Using a disability-adjusted lost life year approach, the burden is estimated at 4-6 life years per person in India alone [12].

Aside from correct breathing and management of stress and respiratory disorders, there are two things we can do with respect to the quantity and quality of oxygen intake. One is to remove from our environment as many noxious substances as possible, and the other is to make small changes to our surroundings to improve our own personal 'air space'. Some ways we can remove noxious substances from our immediate environment include:

1. Giving up smoking (the author is not even pretending this is easy!). Research has shown that smoking cessation with group support is easier than if you try this alone, and you are more likely to be successful if doing it together with others [13].

2. Eliminating the burning of fossil fuels, such as coal and wood where possible, as the smoke produces both carbon monoxide and carbon dioxide, which are damaging to health in the long term [14]. Ventilate homes adequately and find other sources of warmth and cooking facilities such as electricity and piped gas.

3. Keeping homes well ventilated and free from damp as well as vacuuming regularly, or sweeping (with doors and windows open) will help to eliminate dust mites which can aggravate the airways of susceptible individuals [14].

4. Research has shown an increase in asthma, especially in children, is connected to road traffic pollution [15]. Don't go for your early morning run next to the traffic, instead drive to the nearest park and close the car windows if stuck in a jam.

Ways in which we can enhance our personal air space quality include:

1. Getting out into the garden – a walk in a green and peaceful area during the day provides not only relaxation, which in itself is an aid to better breathing [16], but also provides a better quality of air and oxygenation [16].

2. Plants and miniature trees in the office and home environment will aid in the absorption of carbon dioxide and the repletion of oxygen in the air [17], which is especially beneficial in a crowded environment such as an open plan office.

3. Conversely, remove plants from the bedroom at night as this is the time when carbon dioxide is given off, and bring them back again in the morning.

4. Take time to breathe, especially if anticipating a stressful meeting or event. Stand near an open window (preferably next to a garden or lawn) or go for a quick 'walk break' away from the traffic and take ten slow deep abdominal breaths. Deep breathing will aid relaxation and provide more oxygen to the brain, which, in turn, is more likely to be both calming as well as promoting mental alertness [16].

Quick Quiz

Look at the list of items below and decide which of these may be good, not great but passable and not very useful contributions to improving the quality of your personal 'air space'.

1. Underline the items you think are good contributions in green
2. Underline the items you think are not very good but passable contributions in yellow
3. Underline the items you think would not make a useful contribution in red

a.   Sitting near the window in a smoky nightclub

b). Opening the window nearest the garden in a stuffy office

c). Having a pot plant on or near your desk at work

d). Planting a tree in your garden outside the room your family uses the most

e). Deep breathing exercises at your office desk in the coffee break

f). Turning on the air conditioning when a meeting room starts filling up with people

g). Spending the lunch break relaxing with a book on the outside steps of an industrial plant

h). Going for an early morning run along the busy main road

i). Going outside for a walk in the park in the lunch break and doing some breathing exercises in the open air about halfway through

Sunlight, Good and Bad – Maintaining the Balance

The use of sunlight for health (heliotherapy) dates back to ancient Roman and Greek times [18] and has been a treatment option for practising naturopaths since the inception of naturopathic medicine, and the use of sunlight for the treatment of jaundice has recently been medically investigated [19,20]. Some health professionals have for some years been advocating a retreat from sunlight and the use of protecting skin creams even with minimum exposure [21]. Sunlight is a two-edged sword; while we need this essential element for life and health, we also must be cautious about the possibilities and consequences of overexposure to the sun. Sunlight contains several forms of light rays, the best known of which are the UV (Ultraviolet) rays, which are responsible for the production of two essential substances, vitamin D, needed for bone health and strength of the skeletal system and, Serotonin, a neurotransmitter needed for the correct functioning of the nervous system. Sunlight is, in addition, an antibacterial and possibly an anticarcinogenic and has been found to reduce cardiovascular disease [21].

Vitamin D–deficiency rickets is a sunlight deficiency disease. The inability to appreciate the beneficial effect of sunlight for health had devastating consequences for both children and adults for more than 300 years. When it was finally realized that exposure to sunlight could prevent and treat rickets, the recommendation was made that all children be exposed to sensible sunlight in order to maximize bone health [22]. One hour of sunlight exposure can produce the equivalent of 10,000 IU of vitamin D without toxicity, as the process is self-limiting and only the amount of vitamin D that the body can utilise will be produced [23]. Vitamin D is especially important in the prevention of osteoporosis and the strengthening of bone. If maximum bone strength can be attained in the younger years, this serves to lessen the risk of osteoporosis later in life. The elderly and frail who do not go out into the sun are especially at risk of both fracture and the reduction of healing and prolongation of recovery from a fracture [24].

The fortification of milk with vitamin D eradicated rickets as a major health problem, and, therefore, it was thought to have been conquered. Rickets has, however, made an unfortunate comeback [22]. The major cause of rickets in the United States is a lack of appreciation that human milk contains very little if any vitamin D to satisfy the infant's requirement. African American women are often vitamin D deficient, and women who always wear sun protection and only take a prenatal multivitamin are also at a high risk of vitamin D insufficiency [22]. If they provide breast milk to their infant as the sole source of nutrition, the infant will become vitamin D deficient. If the infant is not exposed to sunlight or does not receive a vitamin D supplement, the infant will inevitably develop rickets [22]. The skeletal manifestations of rickets represent only the tip of the vitamin D deficiency iceberg. Vitamin D deficiency in utero and during the first year of life has devastating consequences and may imprint on the child's life, resulting in chronic diseases that will shorten his or her life span. In utero, vitamin D deficiency results in reduced intrauterine long bone growth and slightly shorter gestation [22]. This has been linked to increased risk of osteoporosis and fractures later in life. Children born and raised at latitudes below 35° for the first 10 years have a 50% reduced risk of developing multiple sclerosis later in life [22]. Neonates who are vitamin D deficient during the first year of life are 2.4-fold more likely to develop type 1 diabetes compared with children who received 2,000 IU of vitamin D3 per day [24].

Seasonal Affective Disorder (SAD) is a type of depression that worsens in the winter months and is improved in the summer months with increased exposure to sunlight. Full spectrum light therapy had been seen to be effective for this disorder as it increases the production of serotonin which, in turn, increases the production of melatonin, the neurotransmitter responsible for the regulation of sleeping and waking cycles and mood [25].

There is some controversy surrounding the risk of malignant melanoma (a form of skin cancer) and sunlight exposure [22]. The widespread concern about any direct sun exposure increasing the risk of the relatively benign and non-lethal squamous and basal cell cancers needs to be put into perspective. It is chronic excessive exposure to sunlight and sunburn during childhood that increases the risk of non-melanoma skin cancer. Melanoma, one of the most feared cancers because of its ability to rapidly metastasize before it is obvious to either the patient or physician, has been branded as a sun-induced skin cancer [22]. Most melanomas occur, however, on the least sun-exposed areas. Evidence from several studies has found that the non-exposed surfaces of the skin have a higher incidence of melanoma than the exposed surfaces and it has been reported that occupational exposure to sunlight decreases the risk of melanoma [22].

The 30-year campaign to recommend abstinence from sun exposure has not stemmed the increase in skin cancer incidence. It is curious that in the 1930s and 1940s when children were encouraged to be exposed to sunlight and artificial UV radiation to treat rickets, the incidence of skin cancer did not increase. The peak of skin cancers appeared, however, in the 1970s and, since then, the American Academy of Dermatologists has advised against any therapeutic use of sunlight and maintains that all vitamin D should be obtained from foods and supplements [18]. It is interesting to note that in Turkey, the estimated figures for skin cancers of all types are 5-7% of the total cancer burden; however, 6% of all children under three years suffer from vitamin D deficient rickets [18].

Although sunscreen use is generally advised when exposed to the sun, there is the risk of photo-instability of many of these commercial products, which may lead to a false sense of security at best and an increase in skin damage at worst [26]. Thus, there needs to be a re-evaluation of the beneficial effect of sensible exposure to sunlight as noted by the Australian College of Dermatologists and the Cancer Council Australia, which recommend a balance between avoiding an increased risk of skin cancer and achieving enough UV radiation to maintain adequate vitamin D levels [24].

Based on the current research available, it appears that potential benefits of sunlight outweigh the risks for short term careful exposure [24]. The following guidelines might be useful:

- For infants, 20 minutes per day outdoor exposure to sunlight is adequate [18]
- 15 minutes up to one hour of sun exposure is safe and effective for adults, providing that after the first 15 minutes, a dermatological recommended protective lotion or cream should be applied.
- Frequent short-term exposure is better than single long periods of exposure, and exposure should be built up slowly, beginning with 10 minutes and increasing by 5 minutes every few days.
- Sunning should be avoided between 10.00 am and 3.00 pm

Learning Together

Activity 7.2: Allow yourselves 10 minutes for this activity

  a). As a group, look at each person's exposure to the sun this week, add this up in hours
  b). Multiply by 4 to get the number of 15-minute sun time units.
  c). Divide this figure again by the number of people in your group to t obtain the average sun time units per person.

As 15 minutes of sun exposure (1 sun time unit) gives 10 µg – 40 µg vitamin D (not an exact science), answer the following:

  1. Did everyone get enough sunshine on average?
  2. If not, what foods would you need to have eaten to make up for the lack of sunlight?

Now you should take 5 minutes to discuss the results.

Group Discussion

SEEING THE TREES FOR MORE THAN THE WOODS

In recent years, an increasing amount of research has linked changes in forest cover to several diseases, including some types of yellow fever and others, in particular, parasitic diseases, previously thought to be under control. The role that diminishing forest cover has in the global increase in infectious disease may in some scientist's views be its most direct impact on the health of humanity, albeit not the only impact. In the longer term the intentional deforestation, to provide land for farming, housing and industry as well as the increasing demand for wood products (furniture, timber for building and paper), involved losses of potential sources of medicines, as well as increasing air and water pollution. The most dangerous emissions are those of carbon dioxide and mercury gas into the air. In addition, the concomitant rise in global temperature is permitting certain types of malaria to flourish in areas where it has not existed before moving from tropical to what were once more temperate zones. Extremely worrying to scientists is the loss of the ecosystems that filter toxins from air and water supplies, as well as diluting the strength of the sun's UV rays, thus polluting two of our most basic nutrient resources and changing our exposure levels to the third. Forests purchased for watershed represent the cleanest and most effective use of forest land, as well as providing food sources for people in the form of fruits, nuts, seeds and mushrooms as well as for animal life [17].

Some questions to think about and discuss as a group:
- Given the fact that the following can be grown in a large pot, or in a trough over (or up against) a fence or balcony rail:
    o Miniature plum tomatoes and cherry tomatoes
    o Bay
    o Apricots
    o Lemons, and limes
    o Blackberries and raspberries
    o Green beans and peas

    How much of a contribution do you think you could make to your nutritional status, and air quality in the space that you currently have, be it a garden, patio or balcony?

- What else can you think of that you might do in your own home and garden or on a balcony to contribute to:
    o Your own personal food supplies
    o Your quality of personal air space
    o The amount of clean water you have, or the way in which you currently use water

- Do you think that the act of doing something rather than nothing to improve your nutrition and surroundings will at least make people feel less of a victim and more empowered about their ability to take control of their own situation?

References

1. Whitmire SJ. Water, Electrolytes and Acid-Base Balance. In: Mahan LK, Escott-Stump S, eds. Krause's Food Nutrition & Diet Therapy. 11th ed. Philadelphia: Saunders Elsevier; 2004.

2. Tortora GJ, Derrickson BH. Fluid, electrolyte and Acid-Base Homeostasis. In: Tortora GJ, Derrickson BH, eds. Principles of Anatomy and Physiology. 12 ed. Hoboken New Jersey USA: John Wiley & Sons; 2009.

3. Salfi SF, Holt K. The role of probiotics in diarrheal management. *Holist Nurs Pract* 2012; **26**(3): 142-9.

4. Jennings A, Abdelhamid A, Bunn DK, et al. Water-loss (intracellular) dehydration assessed using urinary tests: how well do they work? Diagnostic accuracy in older people. *The American Journal of Clinical Nutrition* 2016; **104**(1): 121-31.

5. Azoulay A, Garzon P, Eisenberg MJ. Comparison of the Mineral Content of Tap Water and Bottled Waters. *Journal of General Internal Medicine* 2001; **16**: 168-75.

6. Tortora GJ, Derrickson B. Principles of Anatomy and Physiology. 12 ed. Hoboken New Jersey USA: John Wiley & Sons; 2009.

7. Bradley D. Physiotherapy breathing rehabilitation strategies. In: Chaitow L, Bradley D, Gilbert C, eds. Multidisciplinary approaches to breathing pattern disorders. Edinburgh: Churchill Livingstone; 2002.

8. Crinnion WJ. Environmental Medicine. In: Pizzorno JE, Murray MT, eds. Textbook of Natural Medicine. St. Louis: Churchill Livingstone Elsevier; 2006.

9. Wright RJ, Mitchell H, Visness CM, et al. Community violence and asthma morbidity: the Inner-City Asthma Study. *American Journal of Public Health* 2004; **94**(4): 625-32.

10. Gilmour MI, Jaakkola MS, London SJ, Nel AE, Rogers CA. How Exposure to Environmental Tobacco Smoke, Outdoor Air Pollutants, and Increased Pollen Burdens Influences the Incidence of Asthma. *Environmental Health Perspectives*, 2006. http://dx.doi.org/ (accessed 30th September 2007).

11. Annesi-Maesano I, Hulin M, Lavaud Fo, et al. Poor air quality in classrooms related to asthma and rhinitis in primary schoolchildren of the French 6 Cities Study. *Thorax*, 2012. (accessed 19 October 2012).

12. Smith KR. National burden of disease in India from indoor air pollution. *Periodical of the National Academy of Sciences* 2000; **97**(24): 13286-93.

13. Bauld L, Chesterman J, Judge K, Pound E, Coleman T. Impact of UK National Health Service smoking cessation services: Variations in outcomes in England. *Tobacco control* 2003; (12): 296-301.

14. Lowry S. Sources and effects of indoor air pollution. *British Medical Journal* 1989; **299**: 1388-90.

15. Fergusen EC, Maheswaran R, Daly M. Road-traffic pollution and asthma - *International Journal of Health Geographics*, 2004. http://www.ij-healthgeographics.com/content/3/1/24 (accessed 3 May 2007).

16. Chaitow L. Hyperventilation Syndrome / Breathing Pattern Disorders. In: Pizzorno JE, Murray MT, eds. Textbook of Natural Medicine. 3rd ed. St. Louis: Churchill Livingstone Elsevier; 2006.

17. Taylor D. Seeing the forests for more than the trees. *Environmental Health Perspectives* 1997; **105**(11): 1186-91.

18. Aladag N, Filiz TM, Topsever P, Gorpelioglu S. Parents' knowledge and behaviour concerning sunning their babies; a cross-sectional descriptive study. *Biomed Central Pediatrics*, 2006. (accessed 9 May 2007).

19. Colbourn T, Mwansambo C. Sunlight phototherapy for neonatal jaundice—time for its day in the sun?2018. (accessed 29 August 2018).

20. Slusher TM, Vreman HJ, Brearley AM, et al. Filtered sunlight versus intensive electric powered phototherapy in moderate-to-severe neonatal hyperbilirubinaemia: a randomised controlled non-inferiority trial. *The Lancet Global Health* 2018; **0**(0).

21. Razzaque MS. Sunlight exposure: Do health benefits outweigh harm? *J Steroid Biochem Mol Biol* 2018; **175**: 44-8.

22. Hollick MF. Resurrection of vitamin D deficiency and rickets. *The Journal of Clinical Investigation*, 2006. http://www.jci.org (accessed 9th May 2007).

23. Schauss AG. Suggested Optimum Nutrient Intake of Vitamins Minerals and Trace Elements. In: Pizzorno JE, Murray MT, eds. Textbook of Natural Medicine. 3rd ed. St. Louis: Churchill Livingstone Elsevier; 2006.

24. Holick MF. Vitamin D: importance in the prevention of cancers, type 1 diabetes, heart disease and osteoporosis. *American Journal of Clinical Nutrition*, 2004. http//www.ajcn.org (accessed 6th December 2006).

25. Murray MT, Bongiorno PB. Affective Disorders. In: Pizzorno JE, Murray MT, eds. Textbook of Natural Medicine. 3rd ed. St Louis: Churchill Livingstone   Elsevier; 2006.

26. Gonzalez H, Tarras-Wahlberg N, Stromdahl B, et al. Photostability of commercial sunscreens upon sun exposure and irradiation by ultraviolet lamps. *Biomed Central: Dermatology*, 2007. http://www.biomedcentral.com/1471-5945/7/1 (accessed 10 May 2007).

LEARNING SESSION EIGHT: UNWELCOME GUESTS

Introduction

We share our environment internally and externally with both beneficial and harmful microorganisms. We discuss the co-dependency we have with our environment and, how the surrounding microscopic substances are as much a part of the world as we know it, as we are ourselves. Our bodies play host to many microorganisms, some are external, and some live within us. Like long term guests, some are good to have around, while others overstay their welcome, cause disruption and leave us exhausted. We discuss what the most common bacteria are, and where they come from, which ones are the good ones and which ones are bad. We arrive at our first learning together session where we make some decisions about how to assess what we need to eliminate in our environment and how to do this safely.

This session continues with a review of beneficial bacteria, probiotics prebiotics and synbiotics, what they are, how to obtain them and, as useful additions to our internal environment, how we get them to stay. We then look at fungi, some of which are becoming recognised as potential lifesavers, while others cause disease. Once again, there are mechanisms for keeping those which are welcome and showing the door to those which are not.

The second learning together session looks at how to build up our own resistance to harmful substances before we come to our discussion for the day, natural antibiotics, are they a workable solution or an alternative, but somewhat impractical, approach to disease?

Ice-Breaker Quiz

Let us see how much you already know about the tiny microscopic life forms around us. Look at the following statements and decide which are true and which are false:

T / F

1. All bacteria belong on the outside, and any bacteria inside our bodies will only produce disease. _____

2. Bacteria are tiny organisms, but they can be seen through a microscope _____

3. A high concentration of glucose and a mild acid environment favour the growth of bacteria _____

4. Almost all bacteria require water and warmth for growth _____

5. Pasteurisation eliminates dormant or vegetative bacteria in fluids such as juices and milk _____

6. Sunlight has no effect on the growth of microorganisms _____

7. The yeast used to make bread remains active throughout baking and helps to preserve the bread _____

8. An antimicrobial is a substance that kills or inhibits the growth of most known microbes _____

9. Mushrooms, moulds and yeasts are all examples of fungi _____

10. Viruses, unlike bacteria, are large enough to be seen with the naked eye _____

Ice-Breaker Quiz

Sharing the Environment

Cells are the basic units of any living organism, some of which are comprised of many cells that form tissues and organs, making up whole entities such as plants, animals and humans. These are termed multicellular organisms. Others are made up of only a single cell that has a specific formation and a specialised mechanism of survival. These are termed unicellular organisms. Microbes are organisms that are either unicellular or have such a small number or small size of cells that they can only be seen under a microscope and are commonly termed ***microorganisms***. Whether a life form has only one cell or has many cells, there are certain characteristics that all forms of life have in common [1]:

- They reproduce
- They use food as a source of energy
- They synthesise their own internal structures and substances they need for survival
- They excrete their waste
- They respond to changes in their environment
- Sudden (but infrequent) changes in their hereditary characteristics cause them to mutate

Microorganisms are found everywhere. Air currents carry them from the surface of the earth into the upper atmosphere and via winds from continent to continent. They inhabit the seas, lakes and rivers. There may be billions of them in a teaspoon of soil. It is estimated by scientists that the total mass of microorganisms is as much as 25 times the total mass of animal life on earth. The human body contains 10 trillion cells (10,000,000,000,000,000,000) and 100 trillion microorganisms! Microorganisms play a key role in the recycling of elements in nature. Microbes convert chemicals into substances that either plants or animals can use, thus rendering them less dangerous to the environment. Substances that can be decomposed and acted upon by microorganisms are termed ***biodegradable.*** Substances that are synthetic, such as plastics that are not biodegradable, have become a major concern as they are often a source of pollution [1]. Major groups of microorganisms that we share both our external and internal environment with are [1]:

- Protozoa
- Algae
- Fungi
- Bacteria
- Viruses

Protozoa have only one cell and exhibit animal-like characteristics in that they feed on tiny particles in the environment, do not contain chlorophyll and can move by using either fine hairs (cilia) on the cell surface, to crawl along a surface or a whip-like 'tail' (flagella), to move through a liquid (such as pond water or animal blood). Some protozoa cause diseases; one example is malaria carried from stagnant water in the fluid of mosquitoes and transmitted into human blood through the mosquito's saliva. Others are beneficial, such as those found in the stomach of cattle and sheep that help them to digest their food [1].

Algae are considered plant-like as they contain chlorophyll, obtain their energy by photosynthesis have rigid cell walls. They may consist of only one cell or have many cells and be up to several meters in length (in which case they are no longer microscopic). Algae live in water, and in many cases, they cause problems by excreting toxic elements into the water supply. Some, however, are non-toxic and are sources of agar, which is used to solidify fluids and thicken foods such as ice cream. Others provide the basis for anti-inflammatory drugs [1].

Fungi are similar in some respects to algae in that they have rigid cell walls and may consist of a single cell or several cells that form a plant like structure. Fungi do not, however, contain chlorophyll and do not synthesis energy from sunlight but obtain their food from dissolved nutrients in their environment. Moulds are a type of fungi that have several cells, while yeasts have only a single cell. Larger multicellular fungi include mushrooms and bracket fungi which rely on another structure, such as damp soil and grasses, tree stumps and logs for sources of nutrients [1]. Some are the sources of diseases and others are beneficial, and we will discuss this further on in the learning session.

Bacteria are very simple and lack a nuclear membrane and organised intracellular structures. There are two main groups of bacteria, eubacteria and archaebacteria. Eubacteria may be between 0.5 and 5.0 micrometres in diameter and have a variety of shapes, especially spheres, rods and spirals and exist in pairs, groups of four or clusters. Some have flagella and swim through fluids. Some are important in recycling waste materials and are used in the production of medicines. Others cause diseases such as streptococcal sore throat, tetanus, cholera and tuberculosis. Archaebacteria are noted for their ability to survive in harsh environments, including high levels of salt, acids and high heat [1]. They often live in salt flats and heated pools. We will discuss bacteria in a little more depth in the following section.

Viruses represent the border between living and non-living things. Unlike the microbes discussed above, they are not actually cells but are much smaller and simpler. Viruses are so tiny that they cannot even be seen with a normal microscope but require a special extra-powerful electron microscope to be visible to the human eye. Unlike cells, viruses do not have a proper nucleus and contain only one type of nucleic acid, (either DNA or RNA) not two as would normally be found in a cell. Despite their small size, they can do a lot of damage by inserting themselves into the genetic material of the cell of a plant, animal or human. This changes the way the cell functions and is the cause of the mutation of future cells. Viruses are responsible for diseases such as tobacco mosaic (that attacks tobacco plants), foot and mouth disease, (that attacks cattle), and several human diseases, such as human immunodeficiency virus (HIV); polio, the common cold and strains of influenza, to name a few [1].

Quick Quiz

Let us test your vocabulary when it comes to decreasing or killing certain types of 'germs'. Some of these words are seen on the labels of cleaning products, foods and medicines, and you might know them.

1. The term used for substances that kill microorganisms is:

      A. Microbiological agent

      B. Microbicidal agent

      C. X-Rays

      D. UV Rays   _____

2. The term used for substances that either kill or prevent the growth of bacteria is:

      A. Antibacterial agent

      B. Microbacterial agent

      C. Sterilising fluid

      D. Bacteriostatic agent   _____

3. What is the type of cream used to treat Athletes Foot?

      A. Antibacterial

      B. Anti-inflammatory

      C. Antifungal

      D. Fungicidal   _____

4. Killing all organisms present including any spores is called

      A. Sterilisation

      B. Pasteurisation

      C. Homogenisation

      D. Hydrogenation   _____

Bacteria – The Good, the Bad and the Ugly

Bacteria alone accounts for more than half of the weight of human faeces [1]. Surprisingly enough, of the many thousands of bacteria species that we know about, only a few, in fact, cause disease. This has, however, created the impression that all microorganisms, especially bacteria, are bad, damaging and need to be eliminated, which is far from the truth [1]. Within the gastrointestinal tract, there is a complex community of bacteria in which hundreds of species have been identified. The main components of the intestinal flora are good bacteria, predominantly lactobacillus and bifidobacteria organisms [2].

Very little bacterial action occurs in the stomach due to the presence of hydrochloric acid, which acts as a germicide. The small intestine too is relatively sterile, and the predominance of bacteria resides in the large intestine. Colonic bacteria give rise to the formation of gasses, organic acids and lactic acids [2], as well as decomposing bilirubin and other end products of digestion [3]. In addition, bacteria play a role in the final digestion of nutrients, converting any remaining proteins to amino acids and breaking these down further into the chemical substances that the body can use [3]. Colonic bacteria also play a role in the synthesis of vitamins B12 and K as well as assisting the immune system by controlling and inhibiting the over-colonisation of the toxic acid producing bacteria [2,3].

Sometimes, however, things do go wrong, and the bad bacteria can take over when the normal physical functions of the body are disrupted, or the amount of good bacteria present is insufficient. **Helicobacter pylori** (H. pylori) are the bacteria that colonise the stomach lining when the protective mucous coating of the lining or the endothelial lining itself is weakened [4]. Hydrochloric acid may penetrate the lining, which furthers the damage allowing the bacteria to embed itself [5]. H. pylori is responsible for Type B gastritis, peptic ulcers and is possibly a risk factor for the development of gastric cancer [4-6].

Bacterial colonisation of the intestine with pathogenic (disease-causing) bacteria is not uncommon. Such bacteria include *Clostridium, Escherichia, Klebsiella, Salmonella, Shigella, Campylobacter, Streptococcus, Enterococcus and Staphylococcus aureus*. Rotaviruses can also infect the intestinal tract causing severe diarrhoea. The risk of the disease-causing bacteria taking over and inducing illness is reduced if there are sufficient lactobacilli and bifidobaccili present in the gut [6].

Our skin is our largest bodily organ and our biggest source of defence against invading organisms. The skin protects the body, helps maintain body temperature, excretes waste dissolved in perspiration and provides us with sensory information about the outside world. Of all the body's organs, none is more exposed to infection, disease and injury than our skin. It is vulnerable to the elements and constantly exposed to sun, pollutants and microbes. The skin is a semi-permeable membrane that allows in UV light, air and some topically applied creams and medications and keeps out water and many damaging microbes [3].

If one views the skin, especially the exposed parts of the hands, forearms and face under a microscope, one might be quite shocked at the sight! A close-up picture of the human skin could reveal a whole menagerie of exotic looking insect-like creatures, including some forms of mite, which are far from nice but usually not dangerous. Keratin is the substance that protects the underlying tissue of the skin, and the tightly interlocked keratinocytes (skin cells) resist the invasion of harmful microbes. In addition, Langerhans cells on the surface of the skin alert the immune system to the presence of harmful microbial invaders by recognising and processing them. Should this not be sufficient to deal with a bacterial onslaught, macrophages are a type of immune cell situated just beneath the surface of the skin that engulfs harmful bacteria and viruses that manage to bypass the Langerhans cells [3]. As one ages, the production of Langerhans cells diminishes, leaving the skin more open to bacterial infection. In reality, this means that one has to be more careful about skin hygiene and protection as one grows older [3].

Learning Together

Activity 8.1: Allow about 15 minutes for this activity

In small groups look at the following list of bacteria and decide which you feel should stay and which should go – then re-list them under the appropriate heading. Finally, see if you can between you find a way of safely getting rid of the ones you do not wish to keep.

Klebsiella	Helicobacter pylori
Escherichia	Lactobacillus bifidus
Lactobacillus acidophilus	Lactobacillus rhamnosus
Streptococcus thermophilus	Chlamydia
Salmonella	Clostridium difficile

Stay?   Go?

How might you get rid of or keep in check the ones you do not want?

You might wish to take a few minutes to discuss your answers

Probiotics, Prebiotics and Synbiotics

The term **probiotic** was derived from the Greek, meaning 'for life'. The Food and Agricultural Organisation (FAO) and the World Health Organisation (WHO), have stated that there is adequate scientific evidence to indicate a potential for probiotic foods to be of benefit to one's health. There are specific strains of probiotic bacteria (found in fermented foods, especially dairy products) that have been found to be safe for human use. Probiotics are officially defined as "live microorganisms which, when administered in adequate amounts, confer a health benefit on the host" [6,7].

A comprehensive review of the research on probiotics has demonstrated a relatively small but significant number of areas where there is proven clinical effectiveness [7]. These include benefits to new-born babies and children, where there is a susceptibility to intestinal infection, either due to feeding practices, low birth weight or congenital immaturity of the gastrointestinal system. Probiotics have also been found to reduce the severity and duration of diarrhoeal disorders, especially rotavirus infections [8]. Oral probiotics have been successful in the treatment of bacterial gastroenteritis and in alleviating the symptoms of Clostridium difficile [6].

Some scientists believe that the lack of good intestinal flora might be an underlying cause of certain types of inflammatory bowel disease and in many cases, lack of correct intestinal flora will worsen the problems encountered. Evidence suggests that a combination of strains of lactobacilli bifidobaccili and Streptococcus thermophilus bacteria might alleviate the symptoms of disease. Such a combination has been made commercially available to clinical practitioners [6]. Topically or suppository applied multiple strains of lactobacilli have been found to alleviate post-antibiotic therapy genitourinary problems, especially in women and could contribute to women's health [6]. Furthermore, probiotics have been found to be safe for use during pregnancy [6,9]

In the light of mounting evidence for the clinical benefits of probiotics, some commercial manufacturers make claims beyond the capabilities of the products commercially available to the public [6,9]. For many preparations, research has only been conducted in the laboratory and / or in animals, and much is still required in respect of human trials [6,9,10]. With the increase in resistance to antibiotics, their side effects and the potential benefits of the use of probiotics, future trials and good quality effective products available to the health professional community may mean, for many, the difference between continued suffering and a good quality of life [7,10].

Prebiotics are the precursors of internal intestinal flora that the body manufactures within the mucosa covering the intestinal lumen, known as mucosal-associated flora (MAF)[11,12]. These florae are thought to be important in the resistance of pathogens, control of the inflammatory response and immune system stimulation and may be critical in determining the health of the immune system overall. It has been found that specific components of carbohydrate-rich foods, (oligofructose and inulin)[8] are responsible for increasing the MAF in the gut. Both components resist the effects of pancreatic enzymes and are not digested in the small intestine but arrive in the large intestine intact, and subsequently ferment in the mucosal lining. This process results in the provision of a source of energy for the beneficial MAF [11]. Little dietary change is required as the beneficial amounts of prebiotic substances are relatively small [11], food sources include asparagus, bananas, chicory, honey, Jerusalem artichokes, oats, onions and rye [12].

Probiotic therapy can be enhanced with the concomitant use or combined administration of a prebiotic [7]. Such substances are known as **synbiotics**, although such use is currently in its infancy, advantages have been found in its use in treating ulcerative colitis [13]. Synbiotics have been found to increase and sustain beneficial intestinal flora [14]. Synbiotic therapy is currently 'cutting edge', and few trials exist, however, in the light of the increasing evidence in favour of the use of both probiotics and prebiotics, this may hold promise for the future treatment of gastrointestinal and inflammatory bowel disorders [13].

Quick Quiz

Look at the list of foods on the left and try to decide which of them might contain probiotics, which might contain prebiotics, and which may or may not contain beneficial amounts of either but might be good sources of dietary fibre which benefit intestinal health.

Food	Probiotic Source	Prebiotic Source	Good Source of Dietary Fibre
Natural Yoghurt			
Sauerkraut			
Oats Porridge			
Chicory and Endive Salad			
Steamed Asparagus			
Fresh Fruit Salad			
Cottage Cheese			
Pumpernickel Bread			
Onion and Tomato Salad			
Baked Banana with Honey			
Quark/ fromage frais			
Swiss Cheese on Rye			
Stir Fry with Soy Sauce			
Baked Potato with Sour Cream			
Müsli, Honey & Yoghurt			
Roast Vegetables			
Whole Grain Rice Pilaf			
Maize Meal with Maas			
Whole Wheat Salad Sandwich			

Fungi – What is Normal and What is Not?

Fungi can range from single-celled organisms to large multicellular growths such as the bracket fungi (mushrooms). They do not contain chlorophyll and cannot synthesise their own food with the use of sunlight. Instead, they are purely parasitic, that is, they obtain the nutrients they need from the environment [1]. Many of these we do not need to worry about, and indeed some, (certain varieties of mushrooms) are highly nutritious and beneficial [1].

Mushrooms as food contain high levels of protein and potassium. Maitake mushrooms (Grifola frondosa) have been shown to be rich in beta-glucans and to have immunostimulant activity in mice [15] and extracts of the Coriolus versicolor mushroom has been implicated in improved survival times of gastric cancer patients when combined with conventional therapeutic treatments [16]. Such treatments are promising, however, for the present, experimental and further investigation is obviously required.

Of the fungi that are classified as microorganisms, those that are multicellular and produce tiny filaments, such as moulds and yeasts, concern us the most [1]. Moulds may be present without producing toxins, or they may cause mycoses (infection due to toxins from moulds, and fungi). Diagnosis of a mycosis infection is difficult as it is easy to attribute such infections to other causes but more difficult to attribute symptoms directly to mycosis infections [17]. Fungi are the source of mycotoxins which directly cause disease through food contamination, inhalation or, more rarely, contact. Sometimes the cause of the problem is more indirect and due to toxic metabolites of mycoses. There is little research, however, and the source and exact nature of the mycosis infection is often hard to pin down [17].

Candida albicans (thrush / athletes' foot) is a common opportunistic mycosis infection that takes over when one's natural immunity is impaired, either through illness or malnutrition. The nail bed, mucosa of the mouth and throat, and the genitourinary system are most commonly affected areas [5]. This common infection is aggravated by a diet high in sugar, including sucrose, honey, maple syrup and fruit juices [18]. In addition, some experts recommend that those chronically or frequently affected avoid foods containing live / active yeasts and moulds, such as certain varieties of cheese, and alcoholic beverages [18]. Contrary to popular opinion, however, there appears to be no research advocating discontinuation of bread, in which the yeast is killed using a high baking temperature.

Plant substances have been used for centuries by traditional healers in the treatment of microbial infections; however, to date, there are few controlled trials. In recent years some scientists and traditional healers have worked together on reports of the efficacy and safety of herbal treatments. Increased spending on clinically controlled trials and the commercial availability of safe and effective substances is taking place but might take considerable time [19].

Fungal infections are notoriously difficult to deal with and are often recurrent. In the light of the information available, the best way to deal with unwelcome invaders might be prevention, in the form of boosting one's immunity with a good diet, use of prebiotics and probiotics as well as a good lifestyle management programme. Should an infection ensue, then perhaps the safest and most effective treatment, would be that of a timeously initiated conventional antifungal medication combined with a strict curtailment of simple sugars, a good synbiotic supplement and a focus on preventing a recurrence.

Learning Together

Activity 8.2: Allow approximately 15 minutes for this exercise

Taking the activities of your whole learning group, list the five most important ways in which, together, you feel that you are building resistance to harmful substances:-

1. _____
   _____
2. _____
   _____
3. _____
   _____
4. _____
   _____
5. _____
   _____

After listening to the feedback from all the other learning groups, now list three more things that the members of your group could be doing to increase their resistance to 'unwelcome guests'.

6. _____
   _____
7. _____
   _____
8. _____
   _____

You might wish to take a few minutes to discuss your answers

Group Discussion

NATURAL ANTIBIOTICS – WORKABLE SOLUTION OR IMPRACTICAL APPROACH?

Traditional Medicine and biodiversity conservation encompass a number of relevant and contemporary issues which are becoming increasingly apparent [20], as exemplified by WHO's goal in medicines: "to help save lives and improve health by ensuring the quality, efficacy, safety and rational use of medicines, including traditional medicines, and by promoting equitable and sustainable access to essential medicines, particularly for the poor and disadvantaged" [21]. Probiotics, prebiotics, garlic and several herbs (Echinacea purpura; Baptisia tinctoria; Usnea barbarata; Commiphora molmol, Calendula officinalis, Allium sativum and Salvia officinalis) have been used in the treatment of infections [22]. There is some emerging evidence that supports the use of garlic extracts (Allium sativum) in the mitigation of Helicobacter pylori [4]; however, its use in the treatment of fungal infections was found to be of limited value [23]. In the light of increasing antibiotic resistance, given the fact that the aforementioned remedies will not be a quick fix in a critical situation, what does the group think would be practical, effective and cost-effective?

- Should we place more accent on prevention rather than cure?
- Would it be better if nothing was used unless absolute proof of safety and efficacy is found?
- Does the group think that a long history of safe and effective traditional use is of value and that 'more research' might be a waste of money and would take up valuable time?
- Is there perhaps a place for both conventional and complementary remedies in the fight against bacterial, viral and / fungal infections?

References

1. Pelczar MJ, Chan E, Krieg NR. Microbiology Concepts and Applications. New York: McGraw-Hill; 1993.

2. Beyer PL. Digestion, Absorption, Transport and Excretion of Nutrients. In: Mahan LK, Escott-Stump S (eds). Krause's Food, Nutrition & Diet Therapy. 11th ed. Philadelphia: Saunders Elsevier, 2004.

3. Tortora GJ, Derrickson B. Principles of Anatomy and Physiology. 11th ed. London: John Wiley and Sons Inc; 2006.

4. O'Gara EA, Hill DJ, Maslin DJ. Activities of Garlic Oil, Garlic Powder and their Diallyl Constituents against Helicobacter pylori. Applied and Environmental Microbiology. 2000;66(5):2269-73.

5. Nowak TJ, Handford AG. Pathophysiology: Concepts and Applications for Health Care Professionals. 3rd ed. New York: McGraw - Hill Companies Ltd; 2004.

6. Reid G, Jass J, Sebulsky MT, McCormick JK. Potential Uses of Probiotics in Clinical Practice. Clinical Microbiology Reviews. 2003;16(4):658-72.

7. Conly J. Alpha and omega of microbes. Canadian Family Physician. 2004;50:525-7.

8. Kaplan H, Hutkins RW. Fermentation of Fructooligosaccharides by Lactic Acid Bacteria and Bifidobacteria. Applied and Environmental Microbiology. 2000;66(6):2682-4.

9. Reid G, Kirjaivanen P. Taking probiotics during pregnancy. Canadian Family Physician. 2005;51:1477-9.

10. Reid G. Probiotics to prevent the need for and augment the use of antibiotics. Canadian Journal of Infectious Diseases and Medical Microbiology. 2006;17(5):291-5.

11. Langlands SJ, Hopkins MJ, Coleman N, Cummings JH. Prebiotic carbohydrates modify the mucosa associated microflora of the human large bowel. Gut. 2004;53:1610-6.

12. Beyer PL. Medical Nutrition Therapy for Lower Gastrointestinal Disorders. In: Mahan LK, Escott-Stump S (eds). Krause's Food, Nutrition & Diet Therapy. 11th ed. Philadelphia: Saunders Elsevier, 2004.

13. Furrie E, Macfarlane S, Kennedy A, et al. Synbiotic therapy (*Bifidobacterium longum* / Synergy 1) initiates resolution of inflammation in patients with active ulcerative colitis: a randomised controlled pilot trial. Gut. Volume 54, 2005:242-9.

14. Morelli L, Zonenschain D, Callegari ML, Grossi E, Maisano F, Fusillo M. Assessment of a new synbiotic preparation in healthy volunteers: survival, persistence of probiotic strains and its effect on the indigenous flora. Biomed Central Nutrition Journal. Volume 2, 2003.

15. Adachi K, Nanba H, Kuroda H. Potentiation of host-mediated antitumor activity in mice by beta-glucan obtained from Grifola frondosa (maitake). Chemistry and Pharmacology Bulletin. 1987;35:262-70.

16. Nakazato H, Koike A, Saji S. Efficacy of immunochemotherapy as adjuvant treatment after curative resection of gastric cancer. Lancet. 1994;343:1122-6.

17. Bennet JW, Klich M. Mycotoxins. Clinical Microbiology Reviews. 2003;16(3):497-516.

18. Kroker GF. Chronic Candidiasis and Allergy. In: Brostoff J, Challacombe SJ (eds). Food allergy and intolerance. Philadelphia: W B Saunders, 1987:850-72.
19. Cowan MM. Plant Products as Antimicrobial Agents. Clinical Microbiology Reviews. 1999;12(4):564-82.
20. Alves RR, Rosa IM. Biodiversity, traditional medicine and public health: where do they meet? Journal of Ethnobiology and Ethnomedicine. Volume 3, 2007.
21. WHO. Traditional Medicine Strategy 2002-2005. Geneva: World Health Organisation, 2002.
22. McKenna J. Alternatives to Antibiotics - Chapter 6 Herbal Medicine. Cape Town: Struik Publishers (Pty) Ltd; 1996.
23. Carporaso N, Smith SM, Eng RHK. Antifungal Activity in Human Urine and Serum After Ingestion of Garlic. Antimicrobial Agents and Chemotherapy. 1983;23(5):700-2.

LEARNING SESSION NINE: INTRAPERSONAL AND INTERPERSONAL – KNOWING YOURSELF AND GETTING TO KNOW OTHERS

Introduction

Here we look inside at who we really are, our potential for good and how, if at all, we value ourselves. We cannot expect others to respect who we are and what we have to offer if we have no respect for our own strengths, gifts and services. Much of this depends on whether we know who we are, and importantly what we want from life. We look at how much are we worth to ourselves and ask ourselves what sort of person do we eventually aspire to be? We then look at friendship, and we look at how we can be our own best friend as opposed to our own worst enemy. Meaningful friendships with others develop from a place of self-respect and acknowledgement of our own and other people's worth to society. The first learning session looks at our personality traits and explores how we might view these more objectively through the eyes of those around us.

We move on in the next section to discuss the issues of social competence and how this arises, as well as social capital and the benefits we receive from others around us. We look at the value of a supporting and caring friendship with others and ask ourselves: what is a true friend, and how can we become a true friend to someone else? In addition, we review our interactions with others and the positive aspects of belonging to a group. Lastly, we look at the groups that we might belong to and the relationships that the group members have with one another as part of a successful democratic community.

Our second learning together session looks at how we interact in a group and our ability to allow each member to exercise their personal strengths. The discussion of the day revolves around leadership: are good leaders, autocrats or diplomats?

Ice-Breaker Quiz

Circle the words in the three groups below that you feel are most appropriate to you

Intelligent	Slow-learner	Dependable	Flaky
Articulate	Quiet	Considerate	Single-minded
Capable	Clumsy	Forgiving	Bitter
Practical	Airy-fairy	Sympathetic	Unsympathetic
Determined	Irresolute	Friendly	Aloof
Ambitious	Complacent	Lively	Dull
Confident	Insecure	Sincere	Fickle
Assertive	Aggressive	Likeable	Unpopular
Active	Passive	Outgoing	Introverted

Constructive	Destructive	Cooperative	Obstructive
Systematic	Disorganised	Patient	Impatient
Optimistic	Pessimistic	Trusting	Suspicious
Strong	Reticent	Fair-minded	Blame Gamer
Self-aware	Narcisstic	Diligent	Procrastinatious
Self-possessed	Arrogant	Punctual	Tardy
Self-assured	Boastful	Obedient	Disruptive
Wise	Naïve	Cautious	Impulsive
Brave	Timid	Meticulous	Sloppy

Agile	Klutzy	Sensitive	Insensitive
Attractive	Plain	Approachable	Distant
Graceful	Awkward	Affectionate	Cold
Poised	Wall-flower	Tender	Tough
Resilient	Fragile	Content	Unhappy

(adapted from 'What Sort of Person Am I ?'[1]):

Knowing Yourself and Knowing Your Worth

In order to be true to yourself, you need to know what sort of person you are [1], the self-knowledge that you possess is called 'intrapersonal intelligence', and the ability to use it to your advantage is termed 'intrapersonal skill' [2]. Intrapersonal intelligence helps individuals build accurate mental models of themselves and to make decisions about their lives. A high level of intrapersonal intelligence and the development of intrapersonal skill can help one to capitalise on personal strengths and make decisions and choices that make the best use of these strengths, ultimately making the best of oneself [3].

One also needs to remember that positive qualities are no longer positive when taken to extremes, for example taking pride in one's appearance is a positive attribute, especially when in an interview situation when meeting important people or one's prospective in-laws. If taken to extremes, it can manifest in vanity. While being attuned to other people's impression of you is a good thing, constantly worrying about what others think of your appearance can produce a lot of anxiety [1]. A balanced outlook on life that focuses on identifying, strengthening and utilising positive personal attributes, while keeping in check the more extreme or less productive ones, over the long term results in better mental health and greater happiness and well-being [4].

The ice breaker quiz has no scoring system as there is no right or wrong; it is simply for you to explore yourself as no-one else really knows you as well as you do. The purpose of the exercise is not to find out if you are perfect, near perfect or a total flop, or how you compare on the 'goodness scale' with other people. Instead, this exercise provides the opportunity for you to discover all your varied and diverse qualities. If answered honestly, it will increase your intrapersonal skills and bolster your self-esteem. In this way, you can learn to appreciate the inherent strengths you possess and, identify the areas of your personality, which might benefit from some personal development and positive input [1].

Personal attributes that form your personality are, however, only a part of who you are, the other part, is comprised of what you have learned during your lifetime. This, in turn, is influenced by how you learn. Contrary to popular opinion and previous ways of testing intellect, research scientists have come to appreciate that there are 'multiple intelligences' that spread the type of intellectual skills you might possess, across a spectrum [2,5-7]. This is better appreciated as 'learning styles', which are different for each individual [7]. Everyone will have some ability to acquire knowledge across a spectrum of learning styles, but most people will score high (above 15) for one or two particular learning styles [6]. We will take the opportunity to explore our own learning styles in the 'Quick Quiz' session to follow.

Your personal attributes plus the life experiences, how you have learned from these, and what you can use comes close to making you the person you are. As you can see there is no such thing as a bad learning style or lack of intellect [6,7]; it is more a question of degree of difference from those around us that makes us stand out [1]. Such differences if utilised correctly and put to good purpose, can become major strengths and gifts [1]. This is a fact that we all need to appreciate about ourselves; however, some people can do this more easily than others. Being blessed with genuine self-confidence while not being either boastful or overbearing, is rare. It requires a sense of emotional security and the belief that one can be basically a good person and a worthwhile human being even though one makes their share of mistakes [1].

Some people find it difficult to feel good about themselves or even about others and criticise everyone and everything around them, including themselves. This is termed 'self-effacing' and often undermines both self-confidence and the confidence to engage positively with others or take on new tasks. Positive emotions, however, produce positive thoughts, which in turn produce positive results more often than not [8], in turn, this affects health and increases resistance to disease and overall well-being [9]. If you find it difficult to rate yourself positively, go back to the ice breaker quiz and the following learning styles quiz and ask a close friend to rate you instead. They will pick out your good points because they are your friend, and they have reasons to be your friend; you are valuable to this person. Now see yourself in this other person's light. This will give you an indication of your value to others and allow you to develop more objective self-worth.

Another way of improving one's sense of self-worth is to list all the things you do well. Because one's emotions often override the actual facts and cloud observations both about oneself and others [8], it is best to do this exercise over a period of a few days. In this way, there is time to reflect on the list and recall times when you discovered new strengths and abilities. Taking time will also help to override temporary feelings of elation or depression [8]. Attributes can be small, such as hemming new curtains or hanging pictures, or large, such as the ability to write a new computer programme. One should remember to incorporate both natural gifts such as having a nice smile and things you worked hard to achieve, such as landscaping a garden or learning a new language [1].

What is most important is to focus on what one can do comfortably and not on the things that one would like to do or thinks one can do at a stretch. Keep the list and the mind focussed on the positive, those items that one has achieved and can achieve with ease. Focussing on abilities, strengths, and positive attributes allow the mind to achieve these things mentally. This builds up the ability to keep on achieving, thus rebuilding one's self-esteem and self-confidence. Research has also shown that when one feels good about doing a task, then the attention is more focussed, concentration increases and the ability to do the task well increases, thus building more positive feelings [10].

This is, in fact, how we become good at anything and expert at some things, not by building up our weaknesses but by continually focussing on our strengths [11]. A sense of self-worth generates positive feelings about ourselves, which in turn generates more positive feelings about others [8,12] as well as a better state of health [12,13].

Quick Quiz

This quick learning styles quiz has been adapted from H Gardner's multiple intelligence questionnaire in 'Frames of Mind'[2]. Complete the questionnaire by assigning a numerical value of 0-5 (5 = very like me) to each statement.

1. I work well with my hands and am good at fixing things
2. I have a good sense of direction and rarely get lost
3. I can remember the words to my favourite quotes, songs or poems
4. I am usually the one to sort out arguments in the family or between friends
5. I can explain complex matters simply and clearly to others
6. I manage my workload by finishing one task before starting the next
7. I understand my own feelings, and I know why I behave the way I do
8. I am quite a sociable person and enjoy doing things with groups of friends
9. I learn well by listening to others and attending talks and public meetings
10. I experience changes in mood when listening to certain types of music
11. I learn well from charts, diagrams, posters and video clips
12. I enjoy doing crosswords, puzzles and solving logical problems
13. I am sensitive to the atmosphere in a room and the mood of other people
14. I learn best when I must do something for myself
15. I will learn something new if I can see that it will benefit me in some way
16. If I must concentrate on a task, I prefer to be left alone in a quiet room
17. I can listen to an orchestra playing and pick out my favourite instruments
18. I can easily visualise scenes from my childhood and favourite movies
19. I have a large vocabulary and can express myself easily in words
20. I enjoy taking notes and always find them useful after the event
21. I enjoy a physical activity such as dancing and sports and rarely trip or fall
22. I can make connections between experiences, events or ideas
23. I work well in a team and can expand on other people's ideas
24. I am observant and will often see things that other people overlook
25. I get restless, and I am easily bored with long or repetitive tasks
26. I prefer to work or learn by myself
27. I can play a musical instrument, tap out a beat, or hum tunes to myself
28. I can play around with numbers and enjoy mathematical problems

SCORING KEY

LEARNING STYLE	STATEMENTS				TOTAL SCORE
LINGUISTIC	5	9	19	20	
	——	——	——	——	——
MATHEMATICAL AND LOGICAL	6	12	22	28	
	——	——	——	——	——
VISUAL AND SPATIAL	2	11	18	24	
	——	——	——	——	——
MUSICAL	3	10	17	27	
	——	——	——	——	——
INTERPERSONAL	4	8	13	23	
	——	——	——	——	——
INTRAPERSONAL	7	15	16	26	
	——	——	——	——	——
KINAESTHETIC	1	14	21	25	
	——	——	——	——	——

Any score above 15 is deemed to be a high score for that learning style. Your highest scores will indicate the medium in which you learn best.

The Value of Friendship

Friendship is not only enjoyable for its own sake but often impacts on both health and problem-solving in other arenas of life. Research has shown that support from a spouse or someone close can buffer the effects of the stress of daily living and major changes in life circumstances [14,15]. The converse might also be true; however, stress is exacerbated when spouses, family and friends undermine one's ability to cope or one's confidence in the belief that the problem will be self-limiting [15]. Thus, it is important to choose friends wisely, and equally important to be supportive and positive as a friend.

If you discovered in the previous section that you are a good team player and are at your best in the company of other people as well as the kind of person who enjoys doing things in groups, then you already know the value of friendships and will possibly have many friends with whom you engage in certain activities. If on the other hand you have a problem with closeness, intimacy and are not a 'group person', this does not mean that you are doomed to a solitary life.

Developing quality friendships and a close, supportive network of friends, along with a sense of community and social stability to some extent, depends on the previous exercise of knowing oneself and developing a positive self-image [16]. Researchers have found that the image one has of oneself carries over into the way others will view an individual over the longer term. This, in turn, will impact on long term social stability, social adjustment and psychological well-being [16]. It seems that being a good friend to yourself makes it easier to attract and sustain quality friendships and, in turn, to be a good friend to others.

Many people, however, find this difficult and often we hear it said of some individuals, and perhaps even feel ourselves, that we can be our own worst enemy. Self-destruction is the worst kind of destruction as we have no-one else to blame. This trait, however, usually stems from a combination of both ignorance of one's inherent strengths and skills and low self-esteem, accompanied by feelings of worthlessness and self-effacement. In extreme cases, this can lead to preoccupation with what one perceives as gross physical imperfection or skills deficit. Low self-esteem and fear of not having friends or being left alone, along with a preoccupation with perceived physical defects, can lead to a form of mental illness known as body dysmorphic disorder (BDD), which requires medical help [17].

Self-harm is a disorder that results from repeated negative thoughts about oneself and the direction of one's life. It usually occurs with prolonged periods of undiagnosed and untreated depression and / or habitual and persistent negativity concerning one's life at present and prospects for future happiness and well-being [17]. This may, in some measure, be alleviated by the previous exercise of listing one's abilities and positive attributes. Do not allow anything adverse or negative on the list and keep the list going, adding one or two things per day, spending time each day, focussing for two minutes on each item on the list and seeing yourself doing each positive thing [1].

Being your own best friend requires time and effort; however, the result is a better and more balanced self-perception and a more positive view on life overall [1]. Such attributes automatically attract others and with an improved sense of self-worth relationships become more satisfying as we see what we can put into them, as well as enjoying the rewards. When we value ourselves, we have more self-respect and engender respect from those around us. This creates a positive cycle of self-worth and self-confidence.

Psychologists have found that placing our values on our inherent strengths and skills and valuing those around us for their individual strengths and skills has other benefits. The focus on inherent traits and learned skills enhances the value of people for who they are, as opposed to what they have. Developing these values deflects us away from valuing material or monetary status. This, in turn, creates fewer material disappointments in life, strengthens marriages and increases long term health and happiness overall.

Learning Together

Activity 9.1: Allow approximately 20 minutes for this exercise.

Go back to the Initial Ice breaker quiz and first list the ten most dominant positive qualities and then the ten you would most like to change.

<u>Positive Qualities</u>   <u>Wish to Change</u>

1.   1.

2.   2.

3.   3.

4.   4.

5.   5.

6.   6.

7.   7.

8.   8.

9.   9.

10.   10

In your learning groups talk to each other for 5 minutes and without revealing anyone's listed items try to ascertain from talking to the other members of the group what the three most dominant positive attributes of each of the other group members are.

1.   1.   1.

2.   2.   2.

3.   3.   3.

Now, find out if the positive attributes that you think you have, are the same as those that others think you have, you might be surprised to find that there are things you can add to your positive list! In addition, you might also find that something you had previously wished to change might be an attribute, that someone else feels is worthwhile keeping.

You might like to take a few minutes to discuss this exercise briefly

The Benefit of Belonging

Abraham Maslow was a psychologist and philosopher that proposed that human beings have a hierarchy of needs. He postulated that basic needs such as food, warmth and shelter had to be met as well as those of safety from harm before social needs could be met. Social needs include those of finding a suitable partner and forming relationships with others, as well as living in family groups and belonging to a socially cohesive network. In turn, these needs, he felt were more essential that the more 'luxury' requirements of social esteem and self-actualisation or spiritual growth [18]. Some people, however, feel that the need for one another is equal to that of food and shelter and the evolutionary requirements were such that, without the ability to gather food and hunt in groups, we could not have survived as a people [19].

Whichever stance we take it is obvious that we are an interdependent and social species. Perhaps the worst deprivation that can be made is not that of liberty, or even food, but of company. Enforced solitary confinement has been known literally to drive people insane and as such is considered so bad that even as a severe form of punishment, it is no longer allowed. The company of others is one of the mainstays of our existence, providing not just simple companionship but the rewards of sharing both good and bad times, of having a conversation, understanding, empathy with and for others and social support. A sense of connection with other people and of being valued as part of a larger social network are intangible but essential rewards that come with a sense of belonging [19].

Social competence is the ability to relate to those around us appropriately and to function well in social groups and society. It is often defined as the ability to 'fit in'. Social competence most commonly arises out of a childhood where parents have provided a haven for the expression of emotion. The child learns that they can express themselves freely without either the fear of rejection or the fear of being allowed to lose control and damage themselves or their surroundings [20].

You cannot alter your past, but you can learn to free yourself from its negative effects and use what you have learned from it positively. One way of doing this is to make the decision that, regardless of what you think of yourself now, or what you believe other people think, you are lovable and valuable. You must work on that belief and constantly remind yourself until you feel it deep down inside [1]. Allowing for and finding an outlet for emotions, while retaining a sense of self-worth, can allow one to re-build social competence even later in life. This has been proven even with the severely depressed person through cognitive behaviour therapy, a form of 'talk therapy that focuses on the individual's recognition of their problems, talking through solutions and, putting these into practice while reducing stress. This type of therapy can assist anyone regardless of their situation to develop and redefine a new social role [21]. In colloquial terms, this results in the ability to re-invent oneself.

As discussed in earlier learning sessions, doing things in groups holds certain benefits in many areas in life from exercise [22,23] and spiritual development [23] to diet [24] and stress management [25]. Creating relationships with friends, family and one's community with or without a high level of social competence results in what is termed social capital [26]. Social capital, like financial capital, provides social resources in times of stress, trauma, personal need and community-wide problems. This type of resource is invaluable when considering those who have disabilities, long term challenges with health and lifestyle and for the elderly, persons living alone as well as single parents and the newly bereaved [26]. This, in turn, brings us full circle to the evolutionary benefits of belonging and the progression of society. Intimate relationships, close family members and colleagues, one works with, all have a role to play in one's social network as do distant relatives and even casual acquaintances. Relationships with others help us define who we are and our ultimate place in the world. In groups, we are greater than the sum of the individual parts.

Quick Quiz

The following multiple-choice statements will help you find out what your personal friendship preferences are [19]: Mark the statements in each category, that are like you:

1a. I find meeting new people exciting
1b. I am not interested in meeting people with very different lifestyles
1c. I usually back away from people who ask me personal questions
1d. I cannot have a meaningful exchange with someone I have only just met

2a. I tend to withhold judgement of others; everyone has something to offer
2b. I can tell whether someone is my type at a glance
2c. I steer clear of those who look as if they have a sob story to tell
2d. I can usually tell if someone is sensitive or not

3a. I am at ease in most social situations and can strike up a conversation
3b. I find it impossible to communicate with those who have different views
3c. I prefer to talk about impersonal issues rather than personal ones
3d. I can communicate freely with people if I know them well and trust them

4a. I like my colleagues and get on well with them
4b. I am friendly with those who think as I do
4c. I get on with my colleagues but have no close work friends
4d. I have one close work friend, and we discuss our problems over lunch

5a. I am happy to chat with most of my neighbours
5b. I socialise with those neighbours whose lifestyle is like mine
5c. I am civil to my neighbours, but I would not ask them in for coffee
5d. I am friendly with those neighbours I have come to know well

6a. I enjoy big celebrations and large dinner parties with lots of new faces
6b. I prefer a garden party for professional associates and close friends
6c. I would like to go clubbing all night with fun people
6d. I enjoy intimate evenings with one or two close friends and good food

7a. I would enjoy a holiday in a beach house with both old and new friends
7b. I would prefer a trip to Italy with friends who share my love of art
7c. I like action and adventure holidays with lots of activities and sports
7d. I would appreciate a remote getaway break with my best friend

8a. My worst nightmare would be being marooned on a desert island

8b. My greatest fear is to be kidnapped by aliens and unable to get home

8c. My idea of hell is an existential soul-searching psychotherapy group

8d. I could not imagine anything worse than being conscripted into the army

Now look at your main choices:

<u>Mostly a's:</u>   You are a probably **people person** with a sympathetic approach who can relate to others across the board. You have a large circle of friends and tend to bring out the best in those around you.

<u>Mostly b's</u>   You tend to seek friendships that **reaffirm** your view of yourself and life generally and socialise mainly with those of the same socio-economic background and people who mirror your talents. Although you can form close friendships, problems arise if your circumstances change.

<u>Mostly c's</u>   You are good fun and probably have a wide circle of acquaintances but are **non-intimate**, you find it difficult to talk about your feelings and may come across as being more confident than you are. In times of trouble, you might find that you are facing problems on your own.

<u>Mostly d's</u>   You invest a great deal in a few close relationships; one good friend easily satisfies your needs. You can open your heart to someone you trust, and in return, you are **empathetic**, loyal and supportive, but if the relationship fails, you might be devastated and find it hard to trust again.

The Power of the Micro-Democracy

You might think that the more one makes one's own decisions, and the greater the amount of autonomous control, the better one's life will turn out. This, however, can truly backfire as decision making, the resultant responsibility that goes with it and the ultimate responsibility for the outcome can be extremely stressful. This can lead to overload resulting in stress, anxiety and illness [17]. At the other end of the extreme, indecision, the anxiety over not being able to make a decision and the resultant regret involved in constant questioning and self-examination over each possible choice can be equally stressful, resulting in an illness known as anxiety neurosis [17].

Decision making is so stressful that many high-level multinational organisations base their pay structure not on the qualifications required for a given position, but on the decision-making responsibilities and the resultant stress that the position entails [27]. This may not be a wise idea in the longer term as stress is one of the major factors in the generation of both psychological and physical illness [28]. Research in the health and social sciences has demonstrated that autonomous decision making and handing down of the resultant instructions, often do not have the desired effect. Far better results are obtained from a process called 'concordance', an agreement reached between two or more parties, not only as to the best way forward but also to the implementation of a set of instructions designed to achieve change [29].

The process of concordance is reached through another process called 'consultation'. Consultation means to seek information or advice from a person who is engaged in the process of giving professional advice to others in a given field [30]. Consultation is different from 'thought showers', which are designed to be creative but abstract; 'buzz groups' which are merely discussions without necessarily having an outcome; or meetings where the person who called the meeting directs its course and has already written the agenda. In group consultation, each person is acknowledged as an expert in that they have unique strengths and abilities as well as different learning styles, in which problems might have solutions that follow different paths. In consultation, there is no agenda; instead, there is instead a single 'purpose' with an expected 'outcome'. The purpose is either to find a solution to a specific problem or to decide on a way forward given a set of circumstances and defined resources. Group consultation has the following attributes [31]:

- Each member of the group is acknowledged as an equal party to the decision-making process.
- The group acknowledges that all skills, experience, past achievements and current abilities, as well as each person's type of intelligence or learning style, is equally valid.
- Each person contributes equally to the discussion and the decision-making process.
- Each person endeavours to find solutions, partial solutions or to make suggestions, that take into consideration the good of the group or even the good of the wider community affected by the decision.

- The outcome and 'domino effects' of each person's suggestions are carefully considered by the group, and no suggestion is entirely 'rubbished'.
- Each member of the group takes equal responsibility for the outcome regardless of whether the outcome would have been their own individual choice or not.
- No-one considers that they have won or lost at the end of the process as the outcome or decision is that of the group, and no individual has the right of ownership of it.

The democratic process that recognises the input and value of everyone on a small group scale can be used in almost any and every situation that requires either decision making or change. In this manner, concordance can be reached, which has the benefits of the mode and extent of implementation being agreed upon by all.

Learning Together

Activity 9.2: Allow 20 minutes for this exercise

The following exercise is adapted from the book 'Make the Right Decision' [32]. You are going to work in small teams of people who feel that they can think things through and come up with a logical and practical solution to a problem (the advisors). The following scenario is for each of the teams to work through:

A group of 5 people are on a hiking trail through a wilderness area, and come to a wide river about 8 meters across, with trees and rocks on either side of the bank. The wooden bridge which was the original river crossing appears to have been badly damaged in a recent storm, and much of it has fallen into the river. As they contemplate how they are going to cross the river, they realise that only one of the group is a strong swimmer. They are equipped with 40 meters of strong climbing rope and a large canvas tarpaulin. They look around them and find four long pieces of broken planking from the bridge (about 1.5 meters long) have washed up on the bank where they are standing. In a nearby rubbish bin, there are four discarded 5-litre cooking oil cans. Each group should decide what their options are using the consultation process outlined in the last section, and should tentatively decide as to what might be the best option to follow.

You may like to take five minutes to discuss the answers.

Group Discussion

ARE GOOD LEADERS AUTOCRATS OR DEMOCRATS?

Often people are categorised as either leaders or followers and leaders themselves are thought of as being individualistic, solitary, decision makers and autocratic and 'loners,' i.e. preferring not only to stand away from a crowd professionally but also not one who socialises with the masses. Companies often seek out those who have leadership skills and go to great lengths to develop such skills. Leaders, lead but do not always mix. They might interact with others but do not always consult with them or take the suggestions of others seriously. The benefits of autocratic leadership are those of expediency, streamlining and quick decision making in a crisis. Democrats are those who value all around them; they work well in groups and are good at consultation. They are good team players; they can lead if necessary but are not always people who can take large amounts of stress or responsibility. Democrats are diplomatic and often avoid making strong statements or taking a defined stance on their own, without support. The benefits of democratic leaders are that of extensive consultation and concordant decision-making. Looking back to the past exercises that we have engaged with, what does the group think of the two styles of leadership?

- What are the short, medium- and long-term benefits of:
    - Autocratic leaders
    - Democratic leaders
- Is one type of leadership more appropriate to modern day requirements than the other?
- Is there a place for both types of leadership in the world according to the needs of the situation?
- Do we place too much emphasis on one style of leadership and undervalue the other?
- What style of leadership do you think will be more beneficial in the future, and how do you envision the development of this type of leadership?

References

1. Kay A, Larter S, Stacy L, Swainson K (eds). Dare to be Yourself. London: Dorling Kindersley; 1995.
2. Gardner H. Frames of Mind: The Theory of Multiple Intelligences. New York: Basic Books; 1983.
3. Harvard. Gardners Multiple Intelligences - Project Summit (Schools Using Multiple Intelligence Theory) <http://pzweb.Harvard.edu/SUMIT/MISUMMIT.HTM>. Accessed 2004 10 April. Harvard Education.
4. Seligman MEP, Parks AC, Steen T. A balanced Psychology and a full life. Philosophical Transactions of The Royal Society. 2004;359:1379-81.
5. Cave J, Doyle R, Kulpinski D (eds). Assess Your True Potential. London: Dorling Kindersley; 1994.
6. Diaz-Lefebvre R. Multiple Intelligences, Learning for Understanding and Creative Assessment: Some Pieces to the Puzzle of Learning. The Teachers College Record. 2004;106(1):49-57.
7. Tanner K, Allen D. Approaches to Biology Teaching and Learning: Learning Styles and the Problem of Instructional Selection - Engaging All Students in Science Courses. Cell Biology Education. 2004;3:197-201.
8. Clore GL, Huntsinger JR. How emotions inform judgement and regulate thought. Trends in Cognitive Science. 2007;11(9):393-9.
9. Segerstrom SC. Optimism and immunity: Do positive thoughts always lead to positive effects? Brain Behaviour and Immunity. 2005;19(3):195-200.
10. Rowe G, Hirsh JB, Anderson AK. Positive affect increases the breadth of attentional selection. Procedures of the National Academy of Sciences. 2006;104(1):383-8.
11. Satterfield J. Happiness Excellence and Optimal Human Functioning. Western Journal of Medicine. 2001;173:26-9.
12. Seligman M. Authentic Happiness. London: Nicholas Brealey Publishing; 2002.
13. Cohen N, Kehrl H, Berglund B, et al. Psychoneuroimmunology. Environmental Health Perspectives. 1997;105(2):527-9.
14. Brock RL, Lawrence E. A Longitudinal Investigation of Stress Spillover in Marriage: Does Spousal Support Adequacy Buffer the Effects? Journal of Family Psychology. 2008;22(1):11-20.
15. Cranford JA. Stress-buffering or stress-exacerbation? Social support and social undermining as moderators of the relationship between perceived stress and depressive symptoms among married people. Personal Relationships. 2004;11(1):23-40.
16. Diehl M, Hay EL. Contextualised Self-Representations in Adulthood. Journal of Personality. 2007;75(6):1255-83.
17. Persaud R. The Mind - A User's Guide. London: Bantam Press; 2007.
18. Maslow AH. A theory of human motivation. Psychological Review. 1943:370-96.
19. Calman C (ed). Enjoy Satisfying Relationships. London: Dorling Kindersley; 1995.

20. Eisenberg N, Cumberland A, Spinrad TL. Parental Socialisation of Emotion. Psychological Inquiry. 1998;9(4):241-73.
21. Forbes EE, Dahl RE. Neural Systems of Positive Affect: Relevance to Understanding Child and Adolescent Depression? Developments in Psychopathology. 2005;17(3):827-50.
22. Epstein LH, Beecher MD, Graf JL, Roemmich JN. Choice of Interactive Dance and Bicycle Games in Overweight and Nonoverweight Youth. Annals of Behavioural Medicine. 2007;33(2):124-31.
23. Gautam R, Saito T, Kai I. Leisure and religious activity participation and mental health: gender analysis of older adults in Nepal. Biomed Central Public Health. Volume 7, 2007.
24. Hulshof KFAM, Siero FW, May JF, DeJong BM. Long term effects of nutritional group education for persons at high cardiovascular risk. European Journal of Public Health. 2004;14(240-245).
25. Chen JH, Gill TM, Prigerson HG. Health Behaviors Associated with Better Quality of Life for Older Bereaved Persons. Journal of Palliative Medicine. 2005;8(1):96-106.
26. Islam MK, Merlo J, Kawachi I, Lindstrom M, Gerdtham UG. Social capital and health: Does egalitarianism matter? A literature review. International Journal for Equity in Health. Volume 5, 2006.
27. Haldane B, Employment Practices of Multinational Blue-Chip Organisations, 2004, received April 2004,
28. Chalmers AH, Blake-Mortimer JS, Winefield AH. The Prooxidant State and Psychologic Stress. Environmental Health Perspectives. 2003;111(1):A12.
29. Bissell P, May CR, Noyce PR. From compliance to concordance: barriers to accomplishing a re-framed model of health care interactions. Social Science and Medicine. 2004;58:851-62.
30. Reader's Digest Wordpower Dictionary. London: The Reader's Digest Association Limited, 2002.
31. Sabet H. From Global Crash to World Identity. New Delhi: Bahá'í Publishing Trust; 2000.
32. Larter S, Swainson K (eds). Make the Right Decision. London: Dorling Kindersley; 1995.

LEARNING SESSION TEN: MASTERING THE MAYHEM

Introduction

Stress has been termed the biggest killer by many health care professionals. Although the word stress does not appear on a death certificate per se, it contributes towards many health care problems and exacerbates a good number of chronic disorders, thereby piling stress on top of stress. This session helps to evaluate the stress levels in one's own life and clarify one's priorities. We review the issue of time and how to prioritise tasks and create order in our daily lives. In our first learning session, we learn how to make decisions effectively, managing our daily tasks without stress.

We then move on to discuss the emergencies, disasters and setbacks that occur in daily living and how to put these into better perspective. We view ways in which we can control the situation, rather than being overwhelmed by it. In addition, we view ways of controlling the impact of adversity, turning down tasks and responsibilities that are beyond our personal resources, without alienating those around us. Finally, we look at coping skills and contingency plans, how to deal with stress without damage and the skill of advance management. In our second learning together session, we look at how to say no, nicely!

It has been said that we are 10% what happens to us and 90% our reaction to it! Our discussion for today is somewhat controversial as in a rapidly globalising society we are no longer unaffected by other people's problems. As many global concerns are coming to the fore, one realises how interconnected we are as a people on a single planet. Must we, however, be a perpetual victim under pressure, or can personal empowerment, contingency plans and coping strategies work to remove the feelings of victimisation and the resultant stress that goes hand in hand with overload and adversity? Today's topical talking point is 'kicking the ASS (All So Stressful!) out of adversity'!

Ice-Breaker Quiz

Let us first evaluate how we are doing regarding our reactions to life and our ability to manage situations. Look at the statements below and rate how they apply to you, using the scores below the smiley faces.

| Always = 5 | Mostly = 4 | Sometimes = 3 | Rarely = 2 | Never = 1 |

After a particularly stressful day, I look forward to relaxing at home.	
If I have a bad experience, I have a strategy for reducing stress.	
If something goes wrong, it usually looks better after a night's sleep.	
I feel that I am generally optimistic and hopeful about the future.	
If a situation does not work out, I feel that it is probably due to an external factor and is no reflection on my ability or personal worth.	
Regardless of the situation, I don't see a reason to lose my temper.	
I don't feel it is my place to put other people in theirs!	
I think some things are just not worth getting angry about.	
I feel it's amazing what 10 deep breaths by the window can do!	
I feel that nothing can happen to me that I cannot cope with if I trust in my own abilities and my faith in a higher power.	
Total Score	

Evaluating Stress

Stress is one of the most commonly used words in the language of medicine, and yet it is also one of the most difficult to define. Many illnesses are said to be due to stress and can manifest not only on a psychological level as mental health problems, such as depression, phobias and insomnia but equally, on a physical level as a major contributing factor in heart disease, stomach ulcers, irritable bowel syndrome and migraine [1,2]. Stress is a physical reaction to an increase in the output of the hormones of the adrenal cortex, resulting in physical and mental chemical and hormonal changes, which are responsible for the noticeable symptoms of stress [1].

Stress as a cause of illness was almost unheard of a century ago and a rare occurrence only 50 years ago. Today the management of stress-related illness is a major medical problem. The correlation between presumably stressful life events and the incidence of disease was noted more than 25 years ago. Stress appears to reactivate latent viral infections and may well have a role in making individuals more vulnerable to new viral and bacterial infections [1]. Stress-related disorders are already a major public health issue in many countries, and the levels of stress and its global prevalence are expected to become increasingly common in the coming decades [3]. The starting point in dealing with stress is to be able to evaluate two things, the first, is how much stress, one is under, and the second, one's reaction to stress. These are, however, not mutually exclusive factors. Research has shown that the greater the perception of stress, the more support we might require in dealing with it [4].

The first question in the ice breaker focussed on whether one looks forward to going home after a stressful day, a seemingly innocuous question but actually a very important one. If you feel under pressure but someone at home or your close environment is undermining either your ability to cope or your own self-worth and self-confidence, both the perception of stress and the susceptibility to illness, as a result, will be greater [4]. The person who looks forward to going home and has support will not be as susceptible to stress [4]. The effect of this is that both the stress itself and the perception of how bad it is is buffered. Therefore, the two really need to be dealt with as an entity, hence the questions we have asked looked at how we deal with situations, or how we perceive them, as opposed to trying to evaluate stress in isolation.

In recent years the cutting-edge science of psychoneuroimmunology has come into its own and research has found the connection between our emotional and psychological states and the sympathetic nervous system, which controls many physiological functions. These functions include the endocrine system and secretion of hormones, the pro-inflammatory cytokines and, most importantly, the immune system [5]. When we are under emotional and psychological stress, these physical systems break down, resulting in increased blood pressure, inflammatory responses, and lack of resistance to bacterial and viral infection [1]. We may think that we are controlling the stress because we get through a situation on a practical level, however, if we are becoming ill, this may be a sign that we are not in control of the situation at all. This should give us the impetus to respond appropriately. Because stress reactions are caused by changes in body chemistry and hormonal output, there are ways in which we can distinguish between a stress-related problem and an organic problem which is not due to stress [2]. Stress reactions include the following:

- The heart beats stronger and faster
- Blood moves from the skin to the muscles so that the person looks pale and feels tense and shaky
- Muscles tense, especially around the neck and back, often causing a headache
- One cannot concentrate, thinking is affected, and the stressed person is easily distracted
- Although exhausting, stress also causes insomnia
- Mental tension and anxiety results, often with no single perceivable cause

Another way of evaluating the stress one is under, and the response we have to it is to look at life in retrospect, over the last twelve months, noting down the periods of illness, decreased levels of productivity, times of feeling 'under the weather' and days away from work due to health-related problems. Then examine what happened in our lives just prior to these events, noting down changes, increased workload, family, personal and relationship problems or societal problems. Four important questions to ask oneself when evaluating one's health are [2]:

- Did I feel under strain and have feelings of being 'stressed' right from the beginning of the health problem?
- Did something big (good or bad) happen in my life just before I had the symptoms of stress?
- Is there something I can identify that starts off the stressful symptoms?
- Can I identify what happens just before the symptoms go away, i.e. what makes them better or makes them disappear altogether?

Finally, we must understand that not all stress is necessarily bad. We all need some change and variety in our lives. Otherwise, life would be very boring, and the lack of stimulation might lead to more self-destructive behaviours to create excitement in life, for example, extreme sports or the use of substances such as alcohol and recreational drugs. Although variety and change can be stressful, whether we suffer the adverse consequences depends, as stated earlier, on our reaction to it. Two factors are important in this respect, firstly the amount of control we have over the source of the stress and secondly, our basic personality and temperament [2]. When we evaluate stress, we need to evaluate these factors as well. External control, where we are forced to do something against our own wishes is usually more stressful than internal control, where we have made the decision ourselves as to how much to change and the method of change. Knowing oneself and one's own reactions is an excellent tool for understanding what the best coping mechanisms might be. We will deal with this more practically, in the final section of this learning session.

The secret of evaluating stress is to decide concomitantly on the level of control we have and the ability to cope. As this is individual, like the ice breaker quiz, we will each do this for ourselves. We will look at 5 areas of our lives and rate four things, the perceived amount of stress, the locus of control, the amount of control and the ability to cope.

Rating Scale 1= Low   6 = High

	A	B	C	D
Area of Stress	**Amount of Stress**	**External Control**	**Internal Control**	**Coping Ability**
Work, Career & Study				
Home & Family				
Outside Relationships				
Resources & Finances				
Environmental Factors				
TOTALS	**A=**	**B=**	**C=**	**D=**

The scoring formula is as follows is: D + (C-B)-A

E.g.:   A = 20 B=24 C= 6 D=18   **Stress = - 20**
        A = 24 B =12 C =20 D = 32   **Stress = +16**

A negative score means that stress is getting the better of you, but a positive score could mean that you are getting the better of stress, alternatively, that you might not have enough excitement in life, the nearer to zero your score, the better the balance.

Organising Chaos

The first thing to do in a situation of apparent mayhem is deciding what comes first. Part of the problem is forgetting the place of values in creating priorities and in prioritising tasks. What does come first? Happy people are happy because their priorities are in place and they can organise time and resources knowing what to let go of and what to keep [6]. When too much value is placed on the smaller, material and status factors, it is generally at the expense of family, home life and health. Two things result from this; the first is that one literally tries to fit far too many tasks within the available time and financial resources, creating more stress than such items are worth. The second is that family support dwindles and health may not be at a level that allows for physiological resilience, creating the ideal conditions for both physical and emotional illness [6].

Values and priorities go hand in hand, what we value we put first, and this forms the basis of our priorities. We, therefore, begin the process of organisation by reaffirming our values and setting our priorities at the correct level to reflect what we value and what we need. By setting priorities, we can allocate our resources to the most important ones, and 'stop sweating the small stuff'! Abraham Maslow proposed a hierarchy of priorities into which we slot our subsections of actual 'tasks' [7]. Although, as spiritual beings, we think that might be the place to begin, the reality is that spiritual endeavours without any thought to physical needs, the requirements of the law and a commitment to our community and the broader society is somewhat ascetic and can be taken to extremes. We need to think about [7]:

- Biological needs (physical well-being): what we need to do for survival
- Security (physical well- being): physical and mental safety from harm
- Social (psychological well-being): moral/ legal commitments to society
- Esteem (psychological well-being): personal development
- Self-actualisation (emotional / spiritual expression): faith and culture

Note that in none of the above-listed items is the fly now, pay later holiday or the latest haute couture fashion. Sometimes we create our own stress by putting a lot of emphasis on what we want as opposed to sitting down and evaluating what we truly need. We are also required to evaluate what will profit us physically, psychologically and emotionally in the future; if we do not, our lives will only revolve around basic needs. Under these circumstances, life will lack any meaningful purpose [2]. Making decisions about our future well-being helps us to define our future goals and make decisions about the current situation [8]. This in itself can help to bring order into one's life by bringing the locus of control into our own arena rather than allowing external circumstances to dictate how our lives run [2].

Once we have defined our values and set our priorities, then we can look at our goals, which will give us insight into and confirmation of our values, provide direction and establish our future priorities. This takes away the fear of the future and relieves the worry we have now about our future wellbeing. It can, however, be very difficult to decide what you really want out of life.

Many people are less than honest with themselves about their real hopes and desires and end up taking a stab in the dark at what might appear to be an obvious solution to their problems. Others don't give themselves a chance but follow pre-conceived or vague ideas. There are, however, some steps one can take to help define goals and set priorities for the future [8]:

- Separate what you want from what you need, then list only those things that fulfil basic needs (such as suitable accommodation / paid employment) and include what would really make you happy (a country cottage / a fulfilling career).
- Visualise your goal and see yourself clearly in that role. This might include the office, hairstyle, clothing, company vehicle that goes with the job or the garden layout, kitchen and décor of your future home.
- Divide the attainment of your goal into short, (1 year) medium (3 year) and long-term (5 year) plans – then plan the short-term step by step and prioritise this with the other aspects of your current life.

Learning Together

Activity 10.1: Allow 20 minutes for this exercise

We are now going to look at our 24-hour day and make some decisions about tasks and an appropriate amount of time to allocate to essential tasks. In addition, we are going to look at our short-term goals, the category of needs they fall into and allocate time to fulfil these goals. We are going to do this in groups to get a better perspective and come to decisions about time management. We will look at what we need for our holistic physical, psychological and spiritual well-being that is truly essential. You need to state the 'other' needs as well as any of the short-term goals that need to be prioritised and allocated time:

Biological needs (physical well-being): what we need to do for survival

Sleep   _____

Nutrition (preparing food and eating)   _____

Exercise   _____

Other:_____   _____

_____   _____

_____   _____

Short term goals:_____   _____

Security (physical well- being): physical and mental safety from harm

Locking doors at night / setting alarm   _____

Dealing with insurance / pension / paperwork   _____

Other:_____   _____

_____   _____

_____   _____

Short term goals:_____   _____

Social (psychological well-being): moral/ legal commitments to society

Commitments to the community   _____

Earning a living   _____

Caring for dependants   _____

Other:_____   _____

_____   _____

Short term goals:_____   _____

Esteem (psychological well-being): that of personal development

Personal and professional development   _____

Other:_____   _____

_____   _____

Short term goals:_____   _____

Self-actualisation (emotional / spiritual expression): faith and culture

Spiritual devotion   _____

Pursuits of artistic expression   _____

Other:_____   _____

_____   _____

Short term goals:_____   _____

You may wish to take a few minutes to discuss this exercise.

Putting Things into Perspective

There are three things we need to get into their correct perspective when managing both our day to day affairs and our crisis situations:

- How essential is this task?
- How large is this problem?
- Can I afford to ignore it?

Perhaps it might be best to deal with the last issue first. When a task appears to be either insurmountable or, we do not wish to face it, we might engage in avoidant behaviour. Avoidant behaviour includes:

- Use of recreational drugs, alcohol or nicotine
- Overuse or prolonged use of medication
- Oversleeping
- Over prioritising another task
- Abrogating responsibility (procrastination)
- Denying the existence of the task or the problem

Deciding on the day to day tasks

In the previous section, when we looked at priorities, we began to deal with prioritising our daily tasks. We need to ask ourselves when we are overloaded:

- Can we find a way of reducing or even eliminating unnecessary items from our lives?
    - Do we have to do this / is it necessary?
    - Is this, in fact, someone else's priority rather than your own?
    - Is this something you feel you must do because you have always done this task?
- Can we delegate anything?
    - Even very necessary tasks do not always have to be done by one or the same person
- Can we share tasks with someone else?
    - Would this be easier, quicker and / or more effective if shared?

Crisis management

When dealing with a problem, one needs to ascertain how this impacts on life's essential tasks and, by extension, our health and well-being. We then need to ascertain the following:

- How big is this really?
- Are we 'sweating the small stuff' or is it really a life-changing scenario?
- Even in a bad situation, we can ask ourselves how permanent is it?
  - Is it self-limiting or life altering?
- Is solving this problem:
  - Only important to ourselves?
  - Important to our immediate family / community?
  - Of national or international importance?
- Do we have to solve it by ourselves?
- Do we have to solve all of it?

Even in a crisis, it is important to ascertain how much help we can rightfully receive. Often, how much one can ask for and who one can ask is a cultural issue, and one also needs to decide if we have appropriate boundaries. If one feels that one really cannot expand one's own boundaries of support, there are other practical solutions:

- Positive psychology, including guided and focussed meditation
- Spiritual support, including prayer
- 'Anonymous' support groups
  - Alcoholics Anonymous/ Al-Anon
  - Narc-Anon
  - Overeaters Anonymous

Management, Damage Control, or Elimination?

There are three ways of coping with stress which look at both the source of stress and the resources available. The first thing one needs to do with the stress is to decide if the source is removable or not. If not, then the first two options of managing one's life around the problem or controlling the resulting damage will be the main strategies employed. If the stress is removable, then one needs to decide upon a timeline and method of doing this. In the latter case, one needs to control the resultant damage and then move on to reducing and / or eliminating the source of the stress.

Managing the effects of stress

The first thing to remember about stress management is that although one needs to make decisions about management oneself, the process does not have to be undertaken alone. Any health care situation, including that of coping with stress, requires support in order to be effective [9]. Research has shown that one of the greatest barriers to self-care in health management is that of a lack of social support and social capital [9]. Most health care practitioners treating stress-related disorders and any other chronic disorder actually welcome the patient's involvement [10]. GP's will generally encourage self-management as long as they are convinced that measures taken are responsible and supported within the patient's own network [10].

Much of our stress occurs at school or work and sometimes an immediate, even if short-term, answer is better than none at all [3]. Research done with high-level executives and overloaded office administrators demonstrated that an easily accessible online health assessment and stress reduction programme was worth engaging with, even if the results were short-term [3]. A six-month trial of a web-based information and monitoring programme that gave instant feedback was given to the employees who could access it 24 hours per day at work and at home. Results showed that information and monitoring built increased self-knowledge and motivation to manage life and work much better, thus reducing the effects of work-related stress [3]. There were significant health gains from this programme that far outweighed any work time lost with its use [3].

With short term and self-limiting stressors, one might try seeing the funny side, if possible. Deliberately looking for the ludicrous and the ability to laugh something off, actually has some proven benefits when dealing with both the magnitude of the stress and the resultant effect [11]. Exercise, massage and aromatherapy, might help with stress management and damage control but require time and investment of money, whereas laughter is an excellent, inexpensive and immediate fix for short term and moderate stress [11]. It is also a good adjunct to other therapies for long-term and life-threatening disorders, as research supports the fact that laughing improves immune function and resistance to disease [11].

Controlling the damage caused by stress

Damaged caused by stress might be physical, resulting in hypertension, heart palpitations and gastrointestinal disturbances, such as irritable bowel syndrome and stress ulcers, or psychological such as sleep disorders and depression. Alternatively, stress might affect a person both physically and psychologically, as seen with depression and panic disorders. Damage control can also be conducted on a physical level or on a psychological level. Both types of control will result in both physical and mental improvement in response to stress [12]. It might not be easy, however, to engage in psychological control initially, if stress itself is making it difficult to concentrate. It is often easier, to begin with physical measures first, and then move on to a combination of physical and psychological methods, to improve one's resilience and mitigate the damage.

Physical measures include various types of exercise, some of which have multiple benefits. Hypertension is a major problem and a precursor of cardiac disease and stroke that occurs with overweight and bad dietary habits. Stress, in addition, will further increase blood pressure, thus predisposing the individual to an even greater risk of a major cardiac event [13]. Although stress management techniques have been used with such problems, it has been suggested that exercise is perhaps most beneficial [13]. This might be because exercise benefits both the stress and the hypertension problems directly [14]. Tension headaches resulting from stress have been successfully reduced with a programme of Tai Chi. Research shows that this not only significantly reduces or even removes the tendency towards tension headaches but has protective effects against future stress and as such acts as both damage control and a stress management technique [15].

Mindfulness-based stress reduction is the next stage of coping. This type of exercise involves measures such as Hatha yoga or breath control [16], and various forms of meditation, such as guided meditation tapes, transcendental meditation (TM) use of biofeedback, hypnotherapy and alternative concentration techniques (such as walking meditation). All of these methods have been proven over a period of time to reduce both the physiological and psychological effects of stress and improve coping skills [12].

Eliminating the source of the stress

This is very much tied in with the exercise we just completed together as well as the previous quick quiz. If we can eliminate some of the stress sources or at least make changes, we need to decide how we are going to do this and when, or over what period of time. This involves some positive decision making, which needs to be viewed from a positive rather than a negative viewpoint. When we look for creative solutions rather than dwelling on the problem we unblock our minds and tend to see things in a more positive light, over the long term this in itself lessens the impact of the stress and results in a clearer mental picture and a better flow of creativity [17].

Quick Quiz

We are now going to look at some of the things we do in life and ask ourselves if these pastimes help us to:

A. Manage stress
B. Control the damage of stress
C. Eliminate stress altogether
D. Be part of the problem rather than part of the solution!

1. Going for a walk in the park during the lunch break at work
2. Taking ten deep breaths by an open window before and after a meeting
3. Watching a late-night action thriller movie after a hectic day
4. Changing your work environment / office to accommodate some plants and a water feature
5. Using an automated timed computer screensaver with soft music and a country scene
6. Joining a yoga class three times per week
7. A regular Saturday night out on the town razzle, that ends up at a popular nightclub
8. Changing your career to a more creative and flexible occupation
9. Taking a good multivitamin supplement and getting a good night's sleep on a regular basis
10. Starting the working day with a 20-minute Tai Chi session
11. Telling your supervisor / mother in law / next door neighbour exactly what you think of them and getting it all off your chest!
12. Changing to a work from home programme and going into the office only for the vital weekly meetings
13. Sharing childminding / carer duties with another person with dependents, so that you can both have an afternoon a week off
14. Ensuring that home/ work time boundaries are strictly in place
15. A fifteen-minute daily mediation at the end of the working day before starting the dinner

Developing Coping Skills and Contingency Plans

Some things we are born with and others we are born with a little of, but when it comes to the more elusive stuff such as happiness and coping skills, we have been duped into thinking that we either have it or we don't, which in fact is not the case at all . Both are learned traits, the difference being the age at which we learn these traits and whether we have done so in a positive or a negative environment. Health, coping skills, positivism and happiness are often linked because physically healthy people who are optimistic, are happier and cope better [17]. They are more likely to require fewer physical or social 'props' and often place a lesser accent and so a lesser dependency on material goods and social status [6]. One hand washes the other when it comes to coping, happiness and health, and often it is difficult to separate their interdependency [5].

The first rule of developing coping skills is to increase your physiological level of health. Being healthy is the first step to being happy, coping with stress and building a contingency plan. Everything is easier when you are healthy or at least in the best physical condition that you can manage under the circumstances. Added to that, there are a few easy techniques one can use as contingencies for both lesser and greater crisis situations. The next is management, damage control or elimination of the sources of stress. Small but significant coping strategies include the use of the elements.

Getting out into the sunshine is a good way of building psychological well-being through the generation of the neurotransmitter, serotonin. Sunlight helps to alleviate seasonal affective disorder and mild depression, as well as chronic pain [18,19]. Walking on the sunny side of the street is another good habit to get into – wear a pair of shades and exercise in the sunshine, as research indicates that the combination is excellent for alleviating depression and building psychological resilience [20]. Taking a walk in green spaces even on a less than sunny day can also help as it not only aids in relaxation but increases the level of oxygen passing the blood-brain barrier allowing for clearer thinking and better perspective [21].

Counting your blessings is not a last-ditch affair if all else fail; it has been found to be a large factor in keeping things in perspective, building coping strategies and increasing subjective happiness. A research intervention that asked people to write down the weeks 'kindnesses' found that kindness built upon kindness. Those who could count kindnesses were more grateful, and in turn became kinder to others, increasing their social competence, this had the effect of building a favourable social network of support, increasing social capital [22].

Contingency planning is the psychological and spiritual equivalent of living within one's means. It involves creating time and resources for yourself and for emergencies. The following are the main aspects of contingency planning:

- Keeping as healthy as possible under the circumstances in which you find yourself.
- Keep up your social life and value friendship, friends are the family you choose for yourself, and you will need them as they will need you in times of emergency and distress.
- Take part in some form of cultural and spiritual activity on a regular basis not only for your own sake but to support others in the group.
- Make a will and ensure that everyone in your family does this, it should be updated every two years, signed and witnessed
- Make sure that you know where to find help in a dire state of emergency, such as:
    - o The Samaritans
    - o Someone who you know you CAN call at 3.00 is
    - o The citizen's advice bureau or the national equivalent of an emergency legal and financial help and advisory service

Learning Together

Activity 10.2: Allow approximately 20 minutes for this activity

Your group should choose one of the following scenarios and then between you come up with a way of turning down this workload / duty or assistance firmly but with kindness and compassion. The scenarios are A-C, and the strategic 'framework to follow' is given below.

A.	A member of your family who has been dependent on welfare assistance, on an on and off basis for several years, has recently been working full time for six months and has bought a rather expensive new car. They have now (and not for the first time), become unable to work and have asked you to take over the car payments for them until they are well enough to return to work, or find another more suitable job. You could afford to do this 'just', and the family member is aware of this, but it means giving up your family holiday and cancelling your sports club / gym membership.

B.	Your boss, who you have worked for and stood by for many years, is going through a tough mud-slinging and emotional divorce, which for various reasons has taken up all their paid leave allowance. This person now feels that they need a break because of the stress, but it involves their taking a month's unpaid leave and reassigning many of their non-executive duties to you. It will also mean that you must rearrange your own leave to cover the necessary duties in their absence and take it when they return. They know that you have not actually booked your holiday, are flexible when it comes to working hours and are not usually stringent when it comes to boundaries and extra work. You are also friends with their spouse and feel that this might be viewed as taking sides, not to mention taking advantage!

C.	Your sister wishes to go away for a holiday after a major illness but does not wish to take her children with her. You have been taking care of her four children while she was ill and for some weeks after. As you are self-employed from home, this has meant that it has been tough for you, both as far as time management and finances are concerned, as you have lost some lucrative work due to the extra child caring duties. As a result, you have had to dip into your hard-earned savings. Your sister feels that as you are at home all day, you can accommodate her easily and are just being 'bloody-minded' in making her wait for a definite answer so that she can go and book her trip.

Work out a way of dealing with the situation using this strategic framework:

- You are most definitely going to turn down the expected assistance and say no.
- You should not say or do anything; however, that makes the other party feel guilty.
- You should endeavour to be empowering rather than sanctimonious about the fact that you would not have such expectations of others.
- You should try to suggest an alternative solution for them
- You should assure them that you are still prepared to support whatever decision they make with empathy and will still be there for them emotionally, even though you are not going to be part of their practical solution.

You may wish to take a few minutes to discuss your answers

Group Discussion

KICKING THE ASS (ALL SO STRESSFUL!) OUT OF ADVERSITY!

Sometimes we are in situations that appear as if our lives are dictated by politics and politicians, the military, the unwelcome laws, rules and regulations and a total disregard for the individual. People seem to have no time for one another, and it may appear as if we live in a 'dog eats dog' society. Do we have to be the perpetual victim of circumstance, or can we take control?

- Can we now see ways of improving our own lives which are within our means and do not add to the workload?
- Are there mechanisms for coping that we had not previously seen and that we could incorporate into our lives using our new-found knowledge?
- Are we using our full potential, or have we left some of it behind in dealing with the tensions of general living?
- Can we find ways to reassign reorganise or re-prioritise to create more time and emotional space for ourselves?
- Do we have more resources than we thought we had?

References

1. Nowak TJ, Handford AG. Pathophysiology: Concepts and Applications for Health Care Professionals. 3rd ed. New York: McGraw - Hill Companies Ltd; 2004.
2. Persaud R. The Mind - A User's Guide. London: Bantam Press; 2007.
3. Hasson D, Anderberg UM, Theorell T, Arnetz BB. Psychophysiological effects of a web-based stress management system: A prospective, randomized controlled intervention study of IT and media workers. Biomed Central Public Health. 2005;5(78).
4. Cranford JA. Stress-buffering or stress-exacerbation? Social support and social undermining as moderators of the relationship between perceived stress and depressive symptoms among married people. Personal Relationships. 2004;11(1):23-40.
5. Ader R, Kelley KW. A global view of twenty years of Brain, Behaviour, and Immunity. Brain Behaviour and Immunity. 2007;21(1):20-2.
6. Easterlin RA. Explaining happiness. Proceedings of the National Academy of Sciences. 2003;100(19):11176-83.
7. Maslow AH. A theory of human motivation. Psychological Review. 1943:370-96.
8. Larter S, Swainson K (eds). Make the Right Decision. London: Dorling Kindersley; 1995.
9. Bayliss EA, Steiner JF, Fernald DH, Crane LA, Main DS. Descriptions of Barriers to Self-Care by Persons with Comorbid Chronic Diseases. Annals of Family Medicine, 2003:15-21.
10. Blakeman T, Macdonald W, Bower P, Gately C, Chew-Graham C. A qualitative study of GPs' attitudes to self-management of chronic disease. British Journal of General Practice. 2006;56:407-14.
11. Payne-Bennett M. Humour and Laughter May Influence Health: In History and Background. Complementary and Alternative Medicine. Volume 3, 2006:61-3.
12. Grossman P, Niemann L, Schmidt S, Walach H. Mindfulness-based stress reduction and health benefits: a meta-analysis. Journal of Psychosomatic Research. 2003;57:35-43.
13. Johnston DW, Gold A, Kentish J, et al. Effect of stress management on blood pressure in mild primary hypertension. British Medical Journal. 1993;306(963-66).
14. Lutack B, Bongiorno PB. The Exercise Prescription. In: Pizzorno JE, Murray MT (eds). Textbook of Natural Medicine. 3rd ed. Volume 1. St Louis: Churchill Livingstone Elsevier, 2006.
15. Abbott RB, Hui K-K, Hays RD, Li M-D, Pan T. A Randomized Controlled Trial of Tai Chi for Tension Headaches. Complementary and Alternative Medicine. Volume 4, 2007:107-13.
16. Chaya MS, Kurpad AV, Nagendra HR, Nagarathna R. The effect of long term combined yoga practice on the basal metabolic rate of healthy adults. Complementary and Alternative Medicine. Volume 6, 2006.
17. Seligman MEP, Parks AC, Steen T. A balanced Psychology and a full life. Philosophical Transactions of The Royal Society. 2004;359:1379-81.
18. Genuis SJ. Keeping your sunny side up. Canadian Family Physician. 2006;52:422-3.
19. Magnusson A. Light therapy to treat winter depression in adolescents in Iceland. Journal of Psychiatry and Neuroscience. 1998;23(2):118-22.

20. Leppämäki S, Haukka J, Lönnqvist J, Partonen T. Drop-out and mood improvement: a randomised controlled trial with light exposure and physical exercise. Bio-Med Central Psychiatry. 2004;4(22).

21. Groenewegen PP, van-den-Berg AE, de-Vries S, Verheij RA. Vitamin G: effects of green space on health, well-being, and social safety. Biomed Central Public Health. Volume 6, 2006.

22. Otaki K, Shimai S, Tanaka-Matsumi J, Otsui K, Frederickson BL. Happy People Become Happier Through Kindness: A Counting Kindnesses Intervention. Journal of Happiness Studies. 2006 7(73):361-75.

LEARNING SESSION ELEVEN: MIND, MENTALITY AND THE MATERIAL

Introduction

In this session, we look at the power of the mind, how our thoughts create emotions which, in turn, create chemical reactions in our body that affect our health and well-being. We have seen the negative aspect of this in the session previously where the mind can create its own stressful situations, which in turn can affect us physically. Here we take an objective scientific look at the effects of thought, with a brief exploration of the sciences of psychoneuroimmunology and neurolinguistic programming. We then move on to look at how emotions affect our judgement and decision making and how we can use our feelings in a positive, constructive way.

In our first learning session, we are going to do a little experiment for ourselves that demonstrates just how powerful our thoughts can be, in a life-enhancing manner. After this, we move on to how our priorities affect our health overall by revisiting the issue of priorities. We look at what we want as opposed to what we have and creative ways for turning what we have into what we want in a positive manner. Finally, we look at the issue of happiness, is it fate or in fact, a psychological trait? Learning to be happy is possible, and we review the guidelines of the positive psychologists.

This brings us to our second learning together session where we are going to constructively learn how to count our blessings in a way in which makes their worth positively tangible. Finally, we come to our discussion of the day. 'The secret' that everyone is talking about, 'an attitude of gratitude,' is this a myth or a magnet for happiness?

Ice-Breaker Quiz

Focus on the picture below for five minutes:

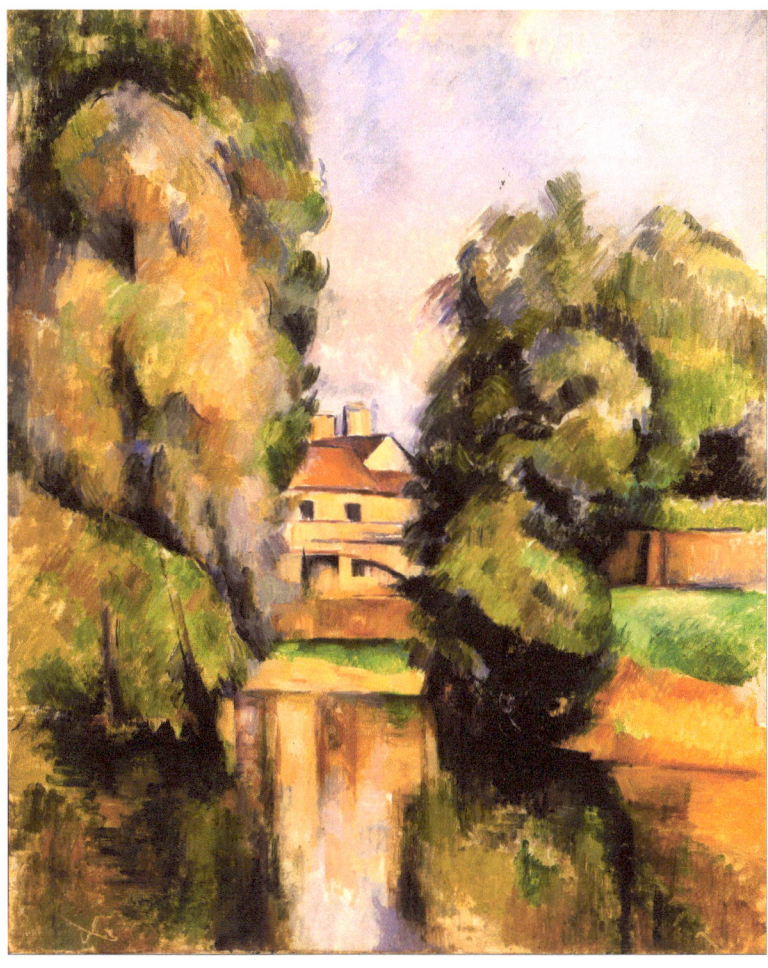

Now cover the picture up and write down the first 20 words that come into your head (we will come back to this):

1. _____
2. _____
3. _____
4. _____
5. _____
6. _____
7. _____
8. _____
9. _____
10. _____
11. _____
12. _____
13. _____
14. _____
15. _____
16. _____
17. _____
18. _____
19. _____
20. _____

Mind and Mentality: The Effects of Thought

Science has built up a store of evidence-based psychological and psychiatric interventions for dealing with mental ill-health, to some extent, at the expense of dealing with mental and emotional well-being [1]. Absence of illness does not, however, equate with optimal health and maximum potential. To be truly healthy and able to optimise and capitalise upon one's physiological and psychological assets, one requires a level of health that goes far and beyond the absence of diagnosable illness. This level of health alone can deal with human poverty on a global scale [2]. Recently, however, this has been addressed in the fields of psychoneuroimmunology, neurolinguistic programming and positive psychology. Positive psychology has to some extent surpassed the other two sciences upon which it was built, dealing more practically with the issue of the use of one's mind to build everyday well-being. It draws upon randomised controlled trials that support the use of exercises that target the use of positive emotions to improve the quality of life [1].

When one is attempting to make changes in life, regardless of whether it is a major change, such as career or home, or a minor change, such as taking up exercise or joining a local organisation, mental attitude is of prime importance. The chances of a successful outcome will be greatly enhanced by an optimistic attitude. This is because, whether we are aware of it or not, the actions of others will sometimes depend on the expectations we have of them, which they may perceive, even if we think that we have hidden our feelings. People will often rise to your expectations in much the same way as they will treat people in the manner that they expect to be treated [3].

If in the previous exercise, your words included calm; tranquil; peaceful, pleasant, or similar words, your general outlook on life is probably one of contentment. If your word list included lonely; isolated; empty, uninhabited or remote, then this is perhaps reflecting how you feel about yourself and your expectations of your present or future home. On the other hand, you might have included words such as adventurous; exciting; invigorating; holiday, retirement or even investment, then your outlook on life and your expectations of it are probably those of positive anticipation. Positive thinkers and optimists tend to see the good things in any situation and pessimists, the challenges or downfalls. This affects one's self-confidence and ultimately how one fares in anything from a job interview to negotiating rental on an apartment [3].

The power of the mind is nowhere more apparent than in the realm of health, on two levels, one is that of psychoneuroimmunology touched on briefly in previous learning sessions, the other that of the placebo effect. The more positive one's mindset and the better one's expectations of the outcome, the less likely one would suffer from a mental health disorder. Similarly, a positive and optimistic outlook on life has been found to have beneficial effects on the risk of cardiovascular disorders, and less chance of rehospitalisation following cardiovascular surgery. The outcome, however, for HIV and Cancer patients is mixed and this has been hypothesised to be due to the fact that both types of disorder themselves are immune system related, and more difficult to treat [4].

The placebo effect is a well-documented phenomenon that involves the strength of the patient's own belief that a particular intervention will work. As the body of knowledge documenting the power of the individual's mind to influence the therapeutic environment and the outcome of illness, conventional medical thinking has begun to change. It is now more readily acknowledged that there is a complex mind-body interaction that influences hormonal and chemical changes which, in turn, influence both the perception of pain and the power to self-heal [5,6]. Even if not effecting a cure, the effects of relaxation and focussed concentration on a more positive endeavour have been found to improve the quality of life for those living with HIV/AIDS [6]. By focussing on positive thoughts and recognising negative thoughts for what they are, unproductive and possibly destructive emotional traits, one can learn to refocus one's mind, thereby regulating and ultimately diminishing unwelcome negative emotional states. Neuro-linguistic programming is a deliberate attempt to tap into the power of the mind by consciously focussing on positive thoughts and breaking the habit of negative thoughts. This has the effect of being more in control of emotion, judgement and the thought process that controls how we feel. Rather than setting up a loop of negativity, there are techniques one can learn that, if practised on a regular basis, can reverse this trend to set up a positive feedback loop [7]. This ultimately will aid in building mental well-being and influencing for the better the physiological processes involved in health and self-healing [4,5].

There have been two pervasive thoughts over the years in the realm of psychology, one of these is that each of us has a 'set point' for happiness, a little like a 'set point' for weight. This theory, however, has little scientific proof. The other viewpoint is that a pervasive or constant state of happiness is somehow not genuine or authentic, and either does not exist or does not count. Psychologist Martin Seligman dubs this the 'rotten to the core' dogma [8]. There have been many self-help books on the power of positive thinking over the past half-century, but the scientific investigation into the realm of positive psychology is relatively new. There is, however, a significant body of evidence emerging for both a palate of techniques with which to implement our new-found knowledge and the evidence for their effectiveness.

Seligman hypothesises that kindness; gratitude, confidence; hope and trust can be developed and used to shore ourselves up against the stresses and strains of both ordinary living and extraordinary problems. Techniques used include some aspects of changing habitual thinking patterns as well as exercising ones core character strengths [8]. Going out of one's way to be deliberately kind, has also demonstrated measurable positive results that affect not only how we feel about ourselves, but how we feel about others and the quality of our lives in general, it seems that kindness begets both more kindness and more happiness [9]. We will explore some of these aspects practically in the quizzes and learning sessions to follow.

Quick Quiz

Laugh and the world laughs with you; laughter has been documented to both relieve stress and lift depression. It has been used in therapeutic healing and pain management [10,11]. The following little quiz is for you to do by yourself but using your ''learning together' group companions. On a scale of 0 (never tense) to 10 (tense on a daily or almost daily basis) rate your overall level of tension considering everyday stress, muscular tension and tension headaches

Thinking back over today, how many times have you laughed, so far?   _____

Now, note how many times you laugh during this learning session   _____

In addition count how many times your companions laugh during the rest of this learning session

Name: _____   _____

Name: _____   _____

Name: _____   _____

Name: _____   _____

Name: _____   _____

1. At the end of the session check with one another that the times you laughed during the session were as many as you thought
2. Check with one another the total times you have each laughed during the day so far
3. Now check the number of times that you laughed against the estimated level of daily tension

Can you now see a connection between daily tension and laughter?

The Power of Feeling

In the realm of cognitive psychology and cognitive behaviour therapy (CBT), the individual learns to recognise and focus on the thoughts that the mind is processing and learns to question their source or validity. It helps in the here and now and in changing thoughts, and thus, changing behaviour as a result [12]. Take for instance the thought of being tired; sometimes we are tired because we have had too little sleep, or we are at the end of a physically demanding day. At other times we simply do not wish to complete a task or face a situation, and we build a psychological resistance towards it that uses up our emotional energy and thus drains the energy required for the task or situation. Other situations that drain our emotional energy are those of jumping to the wrong conclusions, i.e. that something has been stolen from us, whereas, in fact, we have simply mislaid it. Alternatively, we might think that the reason we have not been contacted immediately about the outcome of a job interview, is because we have not got the position, rather than the fact that there is an internal human resources process that must take place.

Unrealistic expectations of ourselves and others, jumping to the worst possible conclusions and trying to force ourselves into a situation, or the performing of an act that subconsciously we do not wish to engage in, can be emotionally (and physically) draining. Persistently doing this can lead to anxiety, impulsive behaviour and a pattern of inappropriate responses to ordinary life situations. If taken to extremes mental health and day to day behaviour are compromised. Talking therapies and focussing on the more positive alternative explanations for both concrete situations and emotional responses can turn this around [12]. Rather than allowing our feelings to manifest in negative thoughts and subsequently negative actions, we have the ability equally to allow feelings to produce energy and galvanise us into more positive behaviour patterns without the inappropriate drainage and subsequent emotional and physical exhaustion [7].

Research shows that human judgement is often the result of emotions and feelings. The more positive the feelings experienced, the more positive the judgement of a situation. This results in more positive behaviour, which, in turn, results in more positive expectations of life. It has been previously assumed that the degree of negative or positive emotions surrounding a task, reflects either how one feels about performing the task or one's own competence to perform it. This, however, has been found to be not quite the case [7]. Pervading feelings in general about oneself, about life and about how the day has run so far, produce a degree of chemical change in the body [13]. The more positive the feelings, the more likely that such changes will result in both the output of epinephrine (a hormone that produces energy) and endorphins (hormones that produce feelings of well-being and diminish feelings of pain) [7,13].

In addition, positive and negative mood states act independently on the judgement and decision-making centres of the brain, affecting how one feels about a given situation. The information processing is faster than the effect of the hormonal changes. This means that firstly, there is a shift in the way in which we judge a situation due to the way the brain works, and messages are sent. Secondly, this is reinforced by chemical changes caused by mood changes. The outcome is that judgement and decision making may not so much be affected by the actual facts concerning the situation, but by the nature of the pervading thoughts and emotional state, we are in, in general [7].

The implication of this ground-breaking research is that such research lends weight to the commonly given advice that one should never make a major decision when ill, overtired, recently divorced or bereaved. Focussing the mind, however, on the most likely positive scenario; making a greater effort to look on the bright side of life; using humour to lighten a mood and counting one's blessings, can have profound effects. Enhancing one's life with sunshine, exercise and stress management can have long-term effects on the judgements we make, our decisions and our future quality of life.

Learning Together

Activity 11.1: Allow approximately 30 minutes for this exercise

Each group is now going to look at the picture below, and in groups, write a short story about the picture, consisting of two sentences to begin, a few sentences about the situation and one or two sentences to end. In total, only a paragraph or, at most half a page, is required. You will then get a chance to read out each group's story.

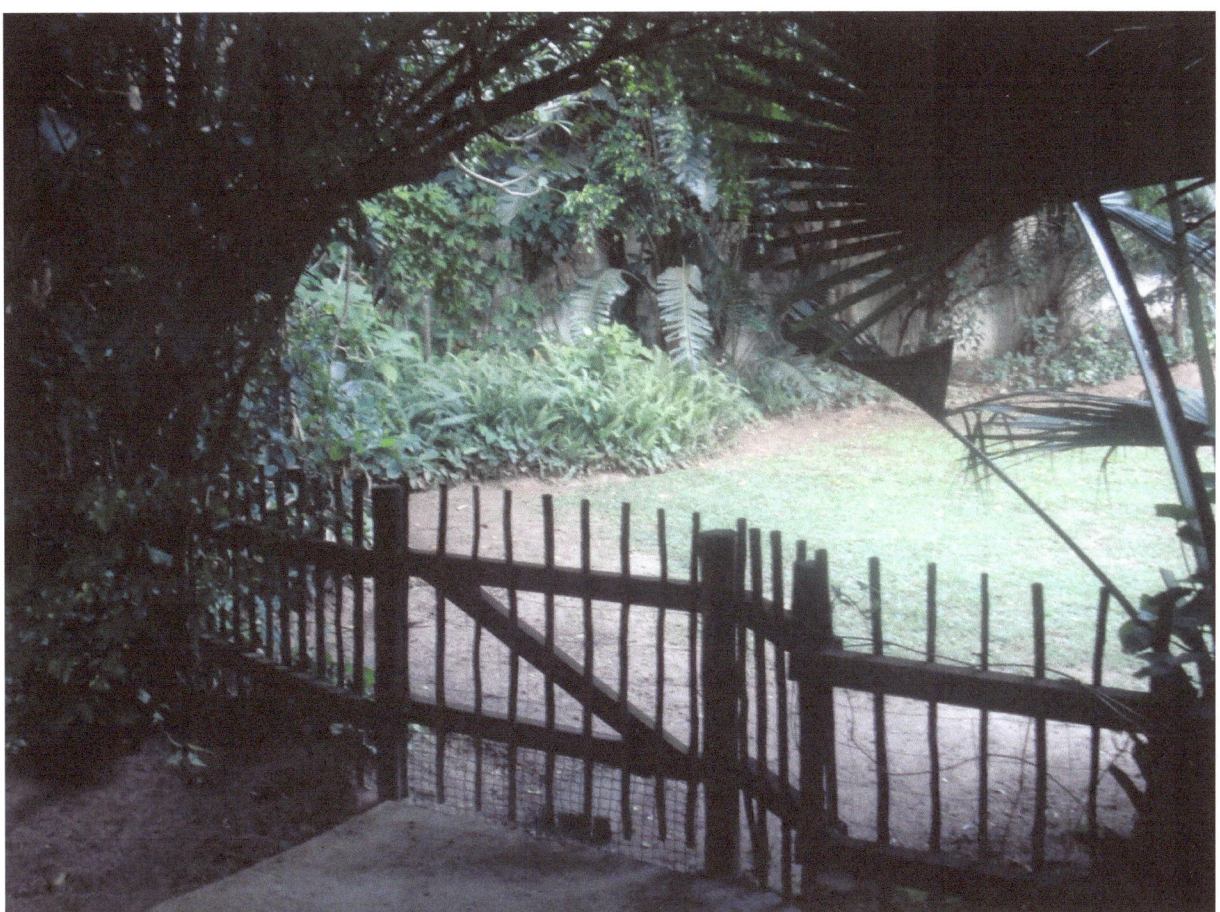

Photograph – Author's own

Now, everyone should make themselves comfortable, take a few deep breaths relax and close their eyes. The facilitator will play a piece of music and read a short, guided meditation, after which, you have the opportunity to re-write your story.

What We Want and What We Have: Our Priorities and Health

In the previous learning session, we touched on priorities and how to allocate time and resources to our goals in life without creating additional stress. To make the best of ourselves and thereby maximise our own potential, we need to be in the best state of health possible, given the assets and considerations we were born with and the opportunities available to us.

In effect, this means that to have the physical and mental well-being, energy and time to get what we want, our goals for health and well-being, need to be compatible with our goals for providing security and fulfilling our biological and emotional needs.

Whether or not we have a current health problem, it is reasonable to make decisions about health improvement, either to improve our current state of health or to lessen the chances of illness in the future. A personal strategy for maintenance and improvement of health is important. Research has demonstrated that when individuals perceive a threat to their well-being, in the absence of a coping response they engage in activities that reduce the fear associated with the threat, rather than dealing with the threat itself [14]. Such strategies include denial or avoidance of the problem or its consequences, such as:

- Pretending that the problem is not at all serious, i.e. It doesn't seem to affect my work / home life / relationships.
- Focussing on the pervasiveness of the problem rather than the outcome, i.e. so many people live with this problem it can't be life-threatening.
- Wishful thinking, i.e. believing that a medical breakthrough will come along and there will be no need to change.
- Fatalism, i.e. believing that the problem runs in the family and the outcome is inevitable regardless of one's own actions.

A good way of setting priorities is to be realistic about where we are in terms of health and define what we wish to aim for. Once we know where we are and have defined where we want to be, we have either consciously or subconsciously stopped denying that there is a problem and lessened the likelihood, that we will avoid it [14]. This strategy makes it easier to face change and take the next step of making the conscious decision to change. This is important as decisions to act, strongly predict that one will change one's health-related behaviour enough to have a positive impact. There is only one more factor involved in this that the locus of control is with oneself, and it is not an enforced intention [15]. As seen from the previous section, the change will be more stressful and less successful if it is in someone else's hands than if one takes the initiative and remains in control of the change process [12,16].

Now we have decided upon what we have, what we want and decided to get what we want; the final step is mapping out a process. This is best done in stages. Trying too hard to get too much too quickly is just setting oneself up for failure. This is the last thing anyone who wishes to achieve a goal wants; however, some people do this as a matter of course. When it comes to change, easy step by step processes are always more successful [17,18]. The following is an overview of how to get the health you want as opposed to the health you have [18]:

1. Assess what you have and evaluate your health, by gathering the information available as to whether you are likely to develop a health-related problem if you do not change any aspect of your lifestyle.

2. Decide on the level of health you would like to have.

3. Decide whether you need to either
   a. Maintain your current lifestyle
   b. Change your current lifestyle

4. List the advantages and considerations of each aspect of change.

5. Decide on a change process for each aspect of health and divide each process into five, six or seven steps.

6. Give each step a date so that the first step is perhaps a week away and small changes are made on a weekly, or monthly basis.

What happens if one relapses? This is normal and expected as any person seeks to change long-standing lifestyle habits. This does not mean that it is back to stage one, but it is possible to re-enter the process at any stage, perhaps, best of all is to re-enter between stages three and six. The goal is to resume some sort of positive action as opposed to having the perfect lifestyle. For a single one-off incident, it is best to simply ignore it and begin the following day as if nothing had gone wrong with the overall lifestyle programme. It is more productive to acknowledge how far one has come along the process and the gains made to date than to focus on the failure [18].

Arguments and self-defensiveness are counterproductive, and one must acknowledge that there are times when one simply cannot do everything. One should focus on what can be done rather than what cannot. For a temporary situation such as a change in working hours, being away from home and out of control of one's situation, it is better to re-date the next step and continue from there on. Treat the relapse in much the same way as one would re-schedule a project plan, work deadline or travel itinerary. For a longer-term problem, focus on one or two small positive changes that can be made and diarise a future date to review the situation [18]. Now we will move on to the final section on creating happiness; when one is happier, everything else is much easier!

Quick Quiz

We will now attempt to measure happiness (even though this is a rather abstract feeling and not an exact measurable commodity). Do you have a positively happy life, or are you in happiness overdraft? First deal with the priority of each area of life (1 = high 8 = low), then how satisfied you are in each area – you may have the same score for more than one category (8=high 1 = low). Now deduct your priority from your satisfaction scores for each category and for your total happiness level.

Area of Life	Priority	Satisfaction	Disparity
HOME			
WORK			
LEISURE			
SPIRITUALITY			
FINANCES			
FAMILY			
HEART			
HEALTH			
TOTAL			_____

Now we will review the issue of whether this is circumstance or perception, can one make oneself happier?

Happiness: Fate or Trait?

Conceptual knowledge that gained through learning is subject to verification in that after receiving a piece of information we then test it, by comparing it to other information we have received or, we review the validity of the source of information. In this manner, we either come to reject it or believe it and assimilate the information, as part of our overall knowledge, beliefs and concepts of life. This is not, however, our only source of knowledge. Emotions and perceptions are also sources of knowledge in that when we feel something, it becomes a personal experience for us, and the truthfulness of that experience cannot be questioned because like sensory perceptions of sight and hearing, it is born of a truth we have experienced for ourselves. In this manner 'feeling is believing' [19].

While the truth of most things can be validated by further knowledge or by the senses (seeing, hearing or touching) affective concepts, the truth of how we feel, cannot be proven by the same method. They are either consensual, in that the same feelings are generated in others by the same experience, or they are self-generated. Self-generated experience includes one's own feelings, and the expression of those feelings as well as the actions that such feelings generate. Negative feelings result in actions of avoidance and positive feelings in actions of approach. When such feelings are appropriate, either because others feel the same way about the same event or because the action they result in is appropriate to the situation, then the feelings are referred to as being congruent with the situation. For instance, it would be congruent to cry at the end of a sad movie and most others watching the same movie would do the same thing. It would also be congruent to laugh at a joke as would most other people hearing it [19].

When feelings are congruent or appropriate to a situation, then the thought processes are fluent, which in neurological terms, means that the brain is processing information quickly, smoothly and correctly. This is important for mental well-being, behaviour and learning, all of which benefit from positive congruent feelings. Research has shown that when feelings are not congruent, such as feeling unhappy in a situation when it would not be appropriate to be unhappy, this results in reduced speed of thought, avoidant behaviour and slower learning [19]. This is an important concept to understand upfront, as it would not be beneficial to learn 'happy behaviour' in a situation that clearly calls for change and / or avoidance. True happiness is not a situation of constant good cheer, as much as one of learning to be appropriately happy and learning how to avoid or change situations which result in constant unhappiness, in a positive and constructive manner [8].

Judgements that are self-serving and which enable people to feel that they are generally honest, hard-working and worthy of life's bounty, are not only ubiquitous but a necessary component of both happiness and health. A positive and happy outlook on life is so necessary to both physical and mental health and well-being that the human being has a regulatory mechanism. Regulation, such as in the operation of a thermostat, involves preservation of an internal state (e.g., generating heat on a cold day to maintain the temperature at a set-point).

The self-serving judgment that controls esteem is an example of a psychological state that is regulated to preserve a stable set point that prevents us from literally going overboard or becoming overly unhappy with ourselves [20]. This is, in fact, regardless of material circumstances.

Self-serving judgements that persuade us that we are not bad people but have unique gifts that are somehow different from others and are worthwhile are supported by modern genetic research. It is no more conducive to nature to create two entities exactly alike than it is to create an entity that is not 'built for success'; hence the dominant genetic traits are generally those that fulfil the requirements of survival and those that subsequently do survive in any given species [21]. Self-belief and belief in one's own worthiness, i.e. that one can and will overcome adversity is therefore built in, as a necessary trait, to ensure survival. Its absence can have dire consequences, but the benefits are perhaps less pressing [20].

Research has shown that people who think that they are unhappy because of material circumstances (such as not owning their own home) and who's circumstances drastically change (through inheritance or winning a lottery) are not, in fact, any happier two years after the event [8]. Despite popular beliefs, salary, age, gender and physical attractiveness have not been found to be predictors of happiness at all [22]. This, according to some psychologists, is due to the 'set point' theory that returns each individual to a homeostatic balance of happiness [20]. If this theory is correct, then happiness has little and quite possibly nothing at all to do with fate.

Martin Seligman, a long-standing researcher in the field of positive psychology, feels that the set-point theory is only part of the happiness equation. Perhaps this is due to the fact that happiness and materialism have less to do with one another than happiness and feelings of both self-worth and personal optimism [8]. The former is concerned with how one views oneself and the latter with one's views of others. Neither outlook on life is carved in stone; both can, in fact, be changed for the better. If this is the case then happiness, regardless of circumstance, can be improved by changing not so much what happens to us, but how we react to it in terms of feelings of self-worth and in terms of how we view our future.

In previous learning sessions, we engaged in exercises that required us to focus on our good points. It is important to keep these in mind and to review them on a regular basis. How we view others, and life's events may need a little creativity if we are to improve this aspect of our lives. One such exercise might appear obvious but is often ignored, and that is reminding oneself of not only one's own good character and worthiness but also the better characteristics of others. Research conducted amongst Japanese students found that happier people were not only more motivated to perform but also recognised and enacted kindness. Asked to record a week's kindnesses, these same students became kinder, more considerate and much happier themselves, they also became more motivated and performed far better [9]. The moral of the story is to count your blessings!

Learning Together

Activity 11.2: Allow yourselves 20 minutes for this exercise

Taking the last week and, including today briefly list below in two columns the kindnesses that you as an individual have performed for others and those that others have performed for you. This does not need to be complex, or magnanimous; it could be as simple as taking a telephone message for someone else or posting your neighbour's letter.

<u>Kindnesses Given</u>   <u>Kindnesses Received</u>

Next, add up the kindnesses given, and kindnesses received, by each member of your learning together group, and divide this by the number in the group to get an average. Now compare your average to the rest of the participant's average and come up with a global group average of kindnesses given and received. Is this more or less than your own personal kindness score? For the next week, keep a daily kindness diary, noting all the little kindnesses you do and those done for you. The idea is to make a conscious effort to better both your own personal kindnesses as well as the average score of kindness given and to be as mindful as possible of those given to each of you.

Group Discussion

AN ATTITUDE OF GRATITUDE, MYTH OR MAGNET FOR HAPPINESS?

Researchers such as Keiko Otaki et al. and Martin Seligman as well as writers such as Rhonda Byrne, and TV personality, Oprah Winfrey are all advocates and personal users of the globally sweeping new psychology of positive thinking. They are, however, not the first; pioneers in this field include the famous entrepreneur Dale Carnegie, the religious multimillionaire super salesman, Zig Ziglar, as well as non-religious scientists such as Candace Pert. Their differences in professional outlook and application of knowledge are vast; however, the thread of truth, in the final analysis, is remarkably similar. See the best in yourself, the best in your surroundings and be grateful! Grateful for what you had, grateful for what you have and grateful for what you are going to get! No-one, however, pretends it is easy, it is not easy, and it takes practice. When life does not turn out well, is it because this theory does not work or because we have simply not had enough practice?

- Does the group think that perhaps we have our priorities wrong when things do not go our way in life?

- Does the group think that, overall, people have too high an expectation when it comes to material wealth and do not look after the physical body or emotional and spiritual side of our lives?

- Alternatively, does the group think that expectations are too low and that some things are simply not a luxury, and life should deliver more than it does?

- Whose fault is it when we are disappointed, other peoples or our own?

- Would counting our blessings and having a more holistic approach to life make us happier?

References

1. Seligman MEP, Parks AC, Steen T. A balanced Psychology and a full life. Philosophical Transactions of The Royal Society. 2004;359:1379-81.

2. WHO. World Health Organisation Report 2004 - Changing History. Geneva: World Health Organisation, 2004.

3. Cave J, Doyle R, Kulpinski D (eds). Assess Your True Potential. London: Dorling Kindersley; 1994.

4. Segerstrom SC. Optimism and resources: Effects on each other and on health over 10 years. Journal of Research in Personality. 2007;41(4):772-86.

5. Bennett P (ed). Placebo and the Power to Heal. Volume 1. Philadelphia: Churchill Livingstone Elsevier; 2006.

6. Cohen N, Kehrl H, Berglund B, et al. Psychoneuroimmunology. Environmental Health Perspectives. 1997;105(2):527-9.

7. Clore GL, Huntsinger JR. How emotions inform judgement and regulate thought. Trends in Cognitive Science. 2007;11(9):393-9.

8. Seligman M. Authentic Happiness. London: Nicholas Brealey Publishing; 2002.

9. Otaki K, Shimai S, Tanaka-Matsumi J, Otsui K, Frederickson BL. Happy People Become Happier Through Kindness: A Counting Kindnesses Intervention. Journal of Happiness Studies. 2006 7(73):361-75.

10. Payne-Bennett M. Humour and Laughter May Influence Health: I History and Background. Complementary and Alternative Medicine. Volume 3, 2006:61-3.

11. Payne-Bennett M, Lengacher C. Humour and Laughter May Influence Health: III. Laughter and Health Outcomes. Complementary and Alternative Medicine. Volume 5, 2008:37-40.

12. Persaud R. The Mind - A User's Guide. London: Bantam Press; 2007.

13. Tortora GJ, Derrickson B. Principles of Anatomy and Physiology. 11th ed. London: John Wiley and Sons Inc; 2006.

14. Norman P, Boer H, Seydel ER. Protection Motivation Theory. In: Conner M, Norman P (eds). Predicting Health Behaviour. Maidenhead: Open University Press: McGraw-Hill Education, 2007.

15. Sheeran P, Milne S, Webb TL, Gollwitzer PM. Implementation Intentions and Health Behaviour. In: Conner M, Norman P (eds). Predicting Health Behaviour. Maidenhead: Open University Press: McGraw-Hill Education, 2007.

16. Bissell P, May CR, Noyce PR. From compliance to concordance: barriers to accomplishing a re-framed model of health care interactions. Social Science and Medicine. 2004;58:851-62.

17. Carels RA, Darby L, Cacciapaglia HM, et al. Applying a stepped-care approach to the treatment of obesity. Journal of Psychosomatic Research. 2005;59:375-83.

18. Snetselaar LG. Counselling for Change. In: Mahan LK, Escott-Stump S (eds). Krause's Food Nutrition and Diet Therapy. 11th ed. Philadelphia: Saunders Elsevier, 2004.

19. Centerbar DB, Clore GC, Schall S, Gavin E. Affective Incoherence: When Affective Concepts and Embodied Reactions Clash. Journal of Personality and Social Psychology. 2008;94(4):560-78.

20. Roese NJ, Olson JM. Better, Stronger, Faster Self-Serving Judgment, Affect Regulation and the Optimal Vigilance Hypothesis Perspectives in Psychological Science. 2007;2(2):124-41.

21. Oppenheimer S. Out of Eden : The peopling of the world. London: Constable and Robinson; 2004.

22. Satterfield J. Happiness, Excellence and Optimal Human Functioning. Western Journal of Medicine. 2001;173:26-9.

LEARNING SESSION TWELVE: FAITH AND FEELING – THE PLACE OF BELIEF AND SELF EXPRESSION IN HEALTH

Introduction

In this final session, we view the presence (or absence), of the divine aspect of our lives and the power of faith. Does this play a role in our lives, and does it affect our health? We review some interesting scientific research on the connection between belief, faith and health. The benefits of faith are not only for those of religious persuasion. Most people have beliefs that are greater than themselves; we attempt to access spiritual strengths that we might not have realised we possess and utilise these, in a creative manner.

In our first leaning session, we look at a compromised and adverse situation and visualise turning this into something better. In this way, we learn the practical techniques of insightful creativity. We then move on to the issue of expressing who we truly are. Lack of opportunities for self-expression can adversely affect our mental well-being, and positive self-expression can additionally be utilised to create a better frame of mind and health. We review ways of doing this that are cost-effective and require next to no talent. Thereafter we look at reason and reality, the issue of whether and if so, why, we self-talk our way out of things when we can self-motivate our way into a better life.

A better life is both reasonable and not unrealistic. We explore this notion before our second learning together session, which looks at creating optimism and selling the benefits on home ground. Finally, we review what we have learned as individuals. We are more aware of the decisions we can make that will make life more productive, healthier and happier for ourselves and for others and as we come to our final discussion, we ask who is really in control of our world?

Ice-Breaker Quiz

Whether we are or are not 'religious' as a learning group, faith and personal belief practices have, throughout history, played a role in politics, culture, development and education. In this session, we look at its role in health. Let us see how much you know about belief per se.

1. Extreme religious practices that call for denial of personal comfort is known as

   A. Asceticism
   B. Sufiism
   C. Yoga
   D. Zen

   Answer: _____

2. Faith-based organised group religious practice is known as

   A. Esoteric practice
   B. Cannon law
   C. Exoteric practice
   D. Catholic practice

   Answer: _____

3. The study of factors that promote health and prevent illness in a population is:

   A. Social medicine
   B. Epidemiology
   C. Population studies
   D. Statistics

   Answer: _____

4. The branch of medicine that deals with the impact of faith on health is:

   A. Psychology
   B. Complementary medicine
   C. Psychoneuroimmunology
   D. Theosomatic medicine

   Answer: _____

Belief and Health

The global population appears to fall into one of three categories as far as belief is concerned; those who believe in a higher power or consciousness, those who believe in themselves and their own innate abilities and those who believe that if they have access to a higher power, they can access their own full capabilities. There is no lack of faith, as much as different expressions of faith, different ways of practising faith and accessing internal potential. So fascinated are we with spiritual consciousness, that regardless of the religious barrenness of scientific belief, scientists have nevertheless devoted an awful lot of time, money and effort in attempting to discover what consciousness is and whether or not we do, or do not, have a soul [1]. For the purposes of this learning session, however, we will not go into such depths of academic argument. Whatever the source of one's own consciousness, faith or self-belief, for practical purposes, we will take the issue of faith in something, (even it is borne of innate self-confidence) as a given.

There are three kinds of impact that faith has on health, one is that of exoteric impact, that is the impact of religious affiliation, fellowship and spiritual support. The second is that of esoteric practice, private spirituality, or the emotional effects of faith on health, as well as the effects of hope and optimism. The third is less tangible and somewhat more difficult to define; it is that of the effect of energy and consciousness on health and healing [2].

There is a significant body of research that supports the fact that exoteric practice, that of community religious worship and regular attendance at a specific place of worship, generates social support or social capital that buffers the effects of stress and isolation [2-4]. The benefits could, in fact, be due simply to the social capital generated, however, it has to be acknowledged that the support of a religious or spiritually based community is likely to be both long term and stable [4]. In addition, is it portable in that physical relocation to another residence might also involve relocation to another, similar place of worship, providing continuation of social capital along with the benefits involved [2]. Alongside this is the beneficial effect of specific health promotion programmes run by faith-based organisations. Such programmes typically include health education; however, many also focus on weight or nutrition, smoking or alcohol cessation. Such programmes are often successful due to the effects of the community support of the participants and have been found to increase the use of screening methods and decrease the incidence of preventable disease [5]. Apart from participation in faith-based health programmes, there are often other activities run by faith-based organisations. It has been found that persons who participate in faith-based cultural and leisure activities have a better quality of life, greater coping skills and less depressive illness [6].

Aside from the preventative benefits, there are benefits to those who already have a life-limiting illness. Religion and spirituality have been found to be connected with a better quality of life for persons living with HIV/AIDS [7]. There are, however, some confounding factors in such aspects of research in that those who are already well enough to attend a place of worship will have greater access to its benefits. As the population of the more affluent countries in the world ages, the concern over the health of the elderly also gathers momentum. In the older population, quality of life is more likely to be linked to the quality of health than any other factor. Such persons may or may not be able to attend a regular religious service or participate in community events due to infirmity. This does not mean that the elderly do not benefit. Spirituality, defined in terms of a sense of meaning, purpose and power from within or from an internal esoteric source rather than specific religious service attendance, has been found to be related to better subjective health and a better quality of life [4,8].

Research into how people recover, and to what extent people recover, from a serious life-threatening illness, involving major surgery and long-term health management, has shown some surprising results. Almost always patients come into two groups, those whose optimism is borne of a long term deep-seated faith that is part of their lifestyle and, the submarine believers who surface only when hit [9]. The former are far more likely to survive, have far less post-operative depression and have far greater post-operative function [9]. The latter suffer greater post-operative depression and function less well having a far worse post-operative function. Unless of course, someone prays for them, in a groundbreaking piece of research on recovery in a cardiac care unit it was found that even in the absence of faith, those who were prayed for recovered more quickly than those who were not prayed for [10].

Simple esoteric faith generates feelings of hope, optimism and positive expectation [4], in this way the impact of spirituality meets with similar results as that of psychoneuroimmunology, which likewise links the emotional aspects of hope and positive expectation to better health outcomes and greater resilience in the face of disease [11]. Research has found that positive thoughts and expectations are closely connected with how we deal with chronic pain and stress. Although to date, management of long-term illness and the accompanying pain has focussed on removing as much stress and pain as possible, there might be benefits in finding ways to increase positive emotions and expectations, which appear to build resilience across the life span [12].

Self-belief, whether borne of religious conviction that one is created in the image and likeness of a higher being, or that each person created is a necessary part of an organic whole, is increasingly deemed necessary to positive emotional, psychological and social development [13]. Researchers have identified that the core qualities of resilience in adult life and the markers of the ability to cope, maintain employment, develop and maintain relationships and to parent successfully, are those of confidence, self-belief, a sense of self-worth and self-respect, as well as a sense of meaning and purpose in life [13]. This is especially the case in the face of high health risk and socio-psychological challenges. Those most likely to overcome challenges and make a success of themselves are not those with extra money, better childhoods, more advantages or necessarily greater family support, but simply the ones who believe they have the ability to succeed and have a higher sense of purpose in life [13,14]. Research into the connection between emotions, expression and health has come up with some interesting facts. Healthy people have a mindset that is characterised by [15]:

- Belief in oneself and one's ability to overcome adversity
- Faith in the future and that it will be better than the past
- Coping mechanisms that are psychological and spiritual as well as practical
- An emotional connection with an unseen power or person
- The ability to be uplifted by music, the arts, or an emotional experience

These attributes are not exclusive to any religion or philosophy; however, all religions and philosophical standpoints encompass the building and maintaining of faith in the future and faith in oneself. This connection between faith and health is also now under the spotlight, and theosophical medicine is not far behind psychoneuroimmunology in becoming a mainstream form of scientific investigation [2]. Churches and faith groups are also becoming more practically involved in building health and well-being. The benefits to the participants of combining practical assistance with faith appear to be outstripping the benefits of either in isolation. Perhaps in the future, health, lifestyle management and faith will come full circle to where it was originally some thousands of years ago, with the added benefits of modern integrative forms of medicine supported by the solidity of independent scientific investigation.

Quick Quiz

We are now going to go back to Maslow's hierarchy of needs and ask you to write or draw in, the items that you feel fulfil each area of personal need in your own life, i.e. food and a home might fulfil biological needs or food, and your spouse and children might fulfil biological needs with your home in your area of security:

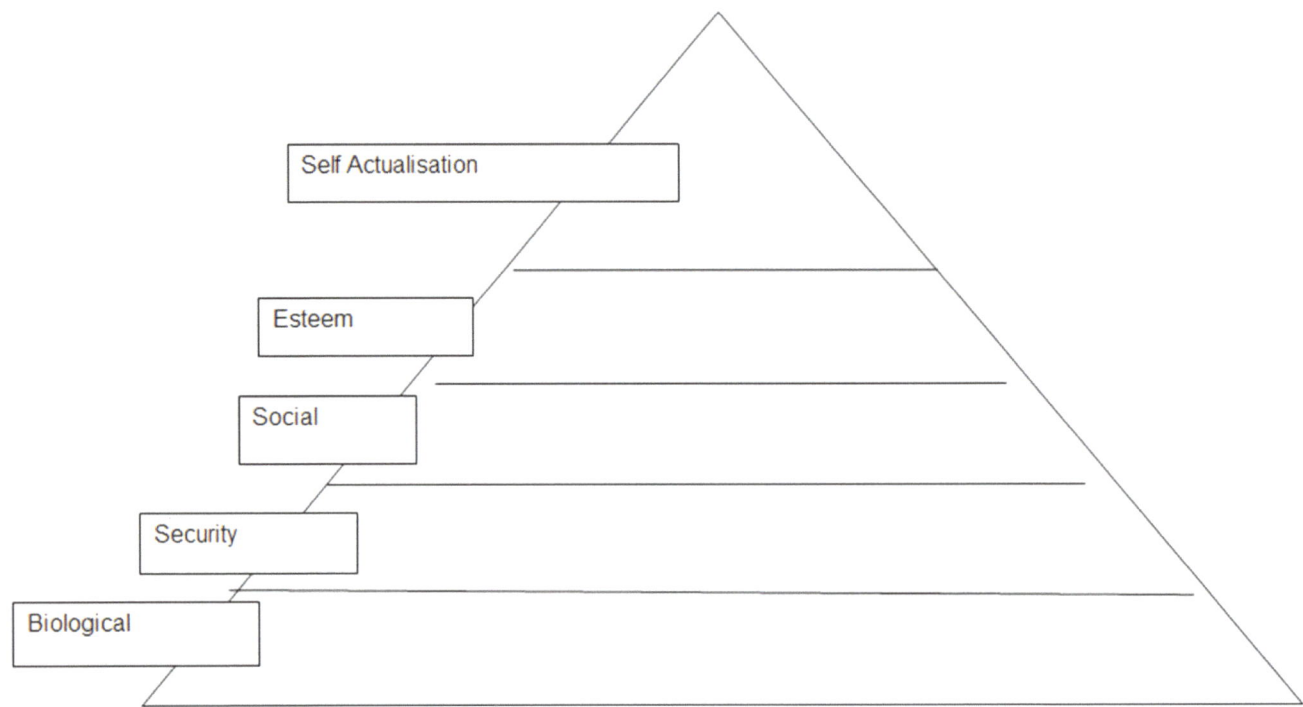

Now rate how full each area is, i.e. if biological needs are fully met; this will be 100%, how full are your esteem and self-actualisation blocks? Lastly, swap your triangle with someone else in your group (this is optional) and see if you can offer one another suggestions for filling the gaps in self-esteem or self-actualisation.

Creative Thought

Creative thought is not a new concept. It has been around in one or another guise for some centuries and, in some respects, it is found in philosophy, the mystical writings of religion and more recently the sciences of neurology, neuroimmunology and behavioural psychology. As we have seen, there is evidence that our thoughts generate emotions, which impact on the autonomic nervous system and the adrenal, hypothalamic, pituitary feedback system. This changes the chemical and hormonal composition in our bodies that, in turn, create conditions of disease, or enhance the capacity of the immune system to heal. Emotions are caused by thoughts that can be brought under control, with practice [15].

The possibility of using our emotions, feelings and thoughts as allies in promoting health and preventing illness is both intriguing and ground-breaking in the overall arsenal of disease prevention. It means that we need to take greater care to understand ourselves, our emotional responses and to begin to reframe how we think about what happens to us. Feelings of loneliness, isolation, alienation and inferiority have been found to impact heavily on mental and emotional well-being. It is, however, these very feelings, alongside those of fear and enmity, that faith often addresses. Ritual, confession, positive emotional arousal and peaceful contemplation may act as conduits for the dissipation of negative emotions and can help us replace these with feelings of personal empowerment [2].

Whether we realise it or not, we are continuously thinking. If we are speaking to someone, we are thinking, as we are if we are listening to someone speak, watching the television or listening to the radio. When we recall memories from the past, we are also thinking and with those memories may come good or bad thoughts, which in turn generate good or bad emotions. For many people, the only time they are not thinking is when they are asleep, but even in the state of sleep, we dream, often of the things we were last thinking about [16].

Thinking is a creative process, like painting or writing, it can be functional, random or controlled. For most people, it is either functional, as in the active concentration involved in thinking through a task at hand, or random, as in the thought processes that go through our mind when viewing a scene, perhaps the news or a traffic jam. Many mindfulness-based relaxation techniques, however, focus on controlled thought, that of actively relaxing by either letting go of negative thoughts and emotions or by enhancing ones of peace and calm.

Active creative thinking involves a process of consciously projecting what one wishes to achieve on to a blank canvas in the mind and then focussing one's thoughts around it [16]. For instance, if one is the sort of person who overreacts to a situation and becomes easily angry, it might be more productive first to see a situation in our mind and then create a scenario where one takes ten deep breaths, relaxes and responds calmly to the situation. The difference between a reaction and a response is that the former is often provocative and confrontational; the recipient of one's anger or reaction might also react creating the scenario for confrontation, stress and adverse physiological responses, such as increased blood pressure and blood glucose levels.

A response, however, arises out of control and calmness; it is self-directed, non-confrontational and rational. Most importantly, there are no adverse physiological consequences arising from a response [15].

Creative thought is different from daydreaming; it is focussed on a single desirable concrete outcome in the future. Creative thought takes what you have and turns it into what you want [16]. Psychologists term this process guided imagery. The few research trials done on guided imagery have found that not only did this reduce headaches and pain, but even in healthy people, reduced overall stress and improved overall mental and physical well-being. It appears that practice is required, however, but participants learned first to conduct the process in groups and then practised at home for up to 20 minutes daily. Those who practised for 20 minutes per day over the course of a year to 18 months benefited from instant relaxation and excellent health [17].

Learning Together

Activity 12.1: Allow approximately 30 minutes for this exercise

The first thing to do is to organise your learning groups into those who are more inclined to use words and those who would like to use pictures. Now each group is required to write down initially a brief scenario that they might have in common and would like to change. (This needs to be something small and specific, such as getting up earlier in the morning, walking on a regular basis, eating cheese and fruit rather than cake and soda, or saying no to an alcoholic drink). We are now going to engage in either one of two activities:

Either:

Re-write the scenario, encasing it in a short story that describes someone successfully carrying out the new action or behaviour and receiving not only the positive results of this action but the rewards that come with it.

Or:

Put together a collage of pictures cut out from magazines of someone successfully engaging in the changed behaviour, the positive outcome and the ultimate goals or rewards.

You may wish to take a few minutes to discuss this.

Expressing Who You Are

Personal expression can be found in many forms, whether it is simply having the freedom of speech, or the ability to express one's deepest inner being through an external medium. Whether we look at this from a human rights standpoint or from a cultural standpoint, the argument for personal expression in the quest for health is vital but not usually discussed. This latter characteristic of health has been used for many years, however, only recently acknowledged as beneficial. Art has been used in health promotion projects and, as an adjunct therapy, it is gaining momentum in the fields of integrated health and psychological well-being. Arts have a shared history with health, but there has been little evaluation outside of the arena of art therapy in the treatment of addictions and long-term chronic conditions. The scientific evidence, however, that links self-expression through the arts with better health outcomes remains elusive [18]. Some practitioners argue that art has a value for its own sake in emotional well-being and should not have to justify itself. Despite the arguments for and against self-expression as a pathway to health, a little light dawns at the end of the long grey scientific tunnel!

Research has found that communities who invest in children's happiness through the provision of the arts, and recreation facilities have healthier children. This held true even when parents were unemployed, or the children came from disadvantaged backgrounds. An investment directly into artistic expression and cultural pursuits for children might well be repaid in the higher health status and lesser need for healthcare in the future [19].

Art has been used in Canadian hospitals for over thirty years, where its use as an adjunct in the treatment of childhood cancer was found to promote pre-treatment relaxation, alleviate fear and allow for personal expression and resolution of fear and anxiety amongst both patients and their families [20]. In addition, self-expression through art can act as a vehicle for adolescents to deal effectively with feelings of depression, academic or social failures and feelings of low self-esteem. In making marks on a paper, forming a collage or moulding a piece of clay or plasticine into the shape of the problem, the problem itself becomes externalised. This externalises the problem, deflecting it away from the individual. The person is then free to be themselves the problem is the external issue and is not any longer a part of who they are. This is a very effective way to separate the difficulties in life from oneself and one's own inherent abilities. Putting something on view with or without having to talk about it can act as an aid in dealing with difficulties [21].

Where some people might baulk at talking therapies with visits to a psychologist, writing might fill the therapeutic gap. If one cannot, or is uncomfortable with verbally expressing feelings, writing it down might be beneficial. The effects of creative writing on health have been found to be quite remarkable. Anything from phantom letters to poetry and prose or short story writing can help not only to manage stress but also in building the capacity for positive psychology, coping and contingency planning. Writing is therapeutic and can aid in building health in the absence of other opportunities for stress management, counselling and support [22].

Music has a power unlike anything else, and its presence is felt across cultures and countries. Music provides a unifying language of expression through happiness and hardship. Music has been found to be motivational, and in the workplace can decrease boredom and increase productivity. Listening to music and making music have been found to increase psychological well-being [23]. Music therapy is an established therapeutic medium that has recently been found to be of use in palliative care, where benefits have included alleviation of pain and stress promotion of energy and lessening of fatigue [24]. Music, in addition, appears to be successful, especially in alleviating depression. Research into the benefits of non-musicians improvising and creating their own music in order to alleviate mental health disorders is currently underway [25], in the meantime, whatever works for you, use it!

Quick Quiz

We have discussed many ways of attaining health through less conventional means throughout this programme. The list on the left represents an assortment of creative activities that one might engage in and on the right, the benefits that one might receive. The objective is to connect the activity to the benefits; it might be helpful to use coloured pencils or pens for this activity.

ACTIVITIES	BENEFITS
Gardening	Promoting sleep
Dancing	Managing stress
Painting	Mental relaxation
Writing poetry	Personal self-expression
Playing a musical instrument	Emotional release
Pottery	Psychological empowerment
Sketching	Mental absorption
Photography	Generating positive feelings
Needlework	Physical relaxation
Listening to music	Keeping physically fit
Storytelling	Physically energising

Reason and Reality

Faced with changes, challenges and possibilities for the future, many people only see the challenge, which in their minds, might loom far larger than the benefits of change. While one might wish for a better life, for some, change is perceived as being more trouble than the benefit might be worth, in addition, a low sense of esteem and confidence may contribute to feelings of inadequacy. Although most people in the world dream of a better life for themselves and can envision what their future might be like if they had a better job, a nicer home, lived in a better area, were physically fitter, or had a better social life, the hurdles along the way are perceived as barriers to the life they want. This translates into 'I cannot… because…'. The betterment is perceived to be imaginary while the obstacles are perceived as being concrete.

The only obstacles that can be proved to exist are those we have overcome. Because we have overcome certain challenges, we know in retrospect that they were challenges and were therefore concrete. The obstacles we think we might face in the future are still in our minds; we do not know whether they are obstacles until we engage in the process of meeting them and attempting to overcome them. The betterment, however, might not be only in one's imagination, the fact that others do have a better home, job, level of fitness or quality of life means that such things are concrete and do in fact exist for some people in some places. This means that they are not unattainable and, given the right circumstances for change, they may not be unrealistic.

The overriding factor in all of this is the recognition of certain thought patterns, the ones that inhibit change and betterment and the ones that empower, guide and promote the use of innate abilities to manage change and create a better lifestyle. This type of internal knowledge of one's own thought patterns and how they work is termed 'self-awareness'. Self-awareness is a key component, alongside the ability to express oneself, regulate one's own thoughts and empathise with people with whom we engage daily of 'emotional intelligence'. Many investigations into this arena believe that the degree of emotional intelligence possessed by an individual is strongly linked to both academic and professional success [26].

It appears that, although hard to measure, assessing the existence of the components of emotional intelligence in both prospective students and job applicants is becoming increasingly popular among academic institutions and large corporations alike. Candidates that know themselves, can express themselves well, and exhibit a certain degree of control over their patterns of thought, managing to keep the damaging ones in check and utilise the empowering ones on a regular basis, are every bit as valuable to some universities and blue-chip companies, as those with good marks and high standards of qualifications. It appears that knowledge and chance are not enough for success, what one does with these attributes and the ability to know how to use one's own thoughts and opportunities in a practical way is the key. Additionally the person who engages in internal politicking is also not necessarily successful; however, those who develop empathy and good relations with others are far more likely to 'get things done' and obtain the resultant recognition for their efforts [26].

Change is not easy, and for many people 'talking oneself out' of acting has resulted in the 'I cannot… because…' pattern of thought. The first two stages of any success, however, are those of, firstly, recognising that the current situation is not what one wants and, secondly, being willing to engage in a change to obtain something one does want. In the previous learning sessions, we have used techniques for getting from one place in life to another, on a practical level as well as at the level of creative visualisation. We are now about to engage in the technique of 'talking oneself in' as opposed to 'talking oneself out' of changes that in the long term, can improve our quality of life. In the learning session to follow, our final group engagement, we will use the technique of changing one's life script alongside an A-D analysis of the situation we wish to change.

Learning Together

Activity 12.2: Take approximately 20-30 minutes for this final learning together session

We are going to do two things in this session. Firstly, we are going to take a typical negative script and rewrite this in a more positive manner using the example given and the template to follow. Secondly, we are going to take the positive script we have created and use the template in the A-D analysis format to see how we can turn a simple act into lifelong success.

Example:
I cannot… *lose weight*, because *I have a sweet tooth* and I cannot *go a whole day without something sweet* because *it is too depressing for me to contemplate not having anything nice*. This means that I cannot *buy nice clothes for myself* because *I am overweight and nice things do not fit me*. I cannot *afford designer plus size clothing* because *I do not have a job*. I cannot *get a job* because *employers do not like overweight employees, and* I cannot *lose weight* because…

Change the script to:
If I changed *the biscuits, I have with tea or coffee for a small piece of fresh ripe fruit* the advantage would be *that I would have something sweet that is healthier and contains less fat, sugar and calories*. If I changed *this pattern of snacking for a few months*, the advantage would be *that I would lose weight, look better and feel better*. If I changed *the biscuits for something equally nice*, the advantage would be *that I would not be depressed about not having something sweet because I would be having something equally nice to eat*. If I changed *my weight and improved my sense of well-being*, the advantage would be *that I would feel good about myself as well as looking better*. If I changed *the way I feel about myself*, the advantage would be *that this would come across in a job interview*. If I changed *my financial circumstances by getting a job*, the advantage would be *that I could earn money for new clothes that would look good on me*. If I changed *my overall appearance and state of health*, the advantage would be etc.

Transposed on to an A-D analysis this looks like the chart that follows:

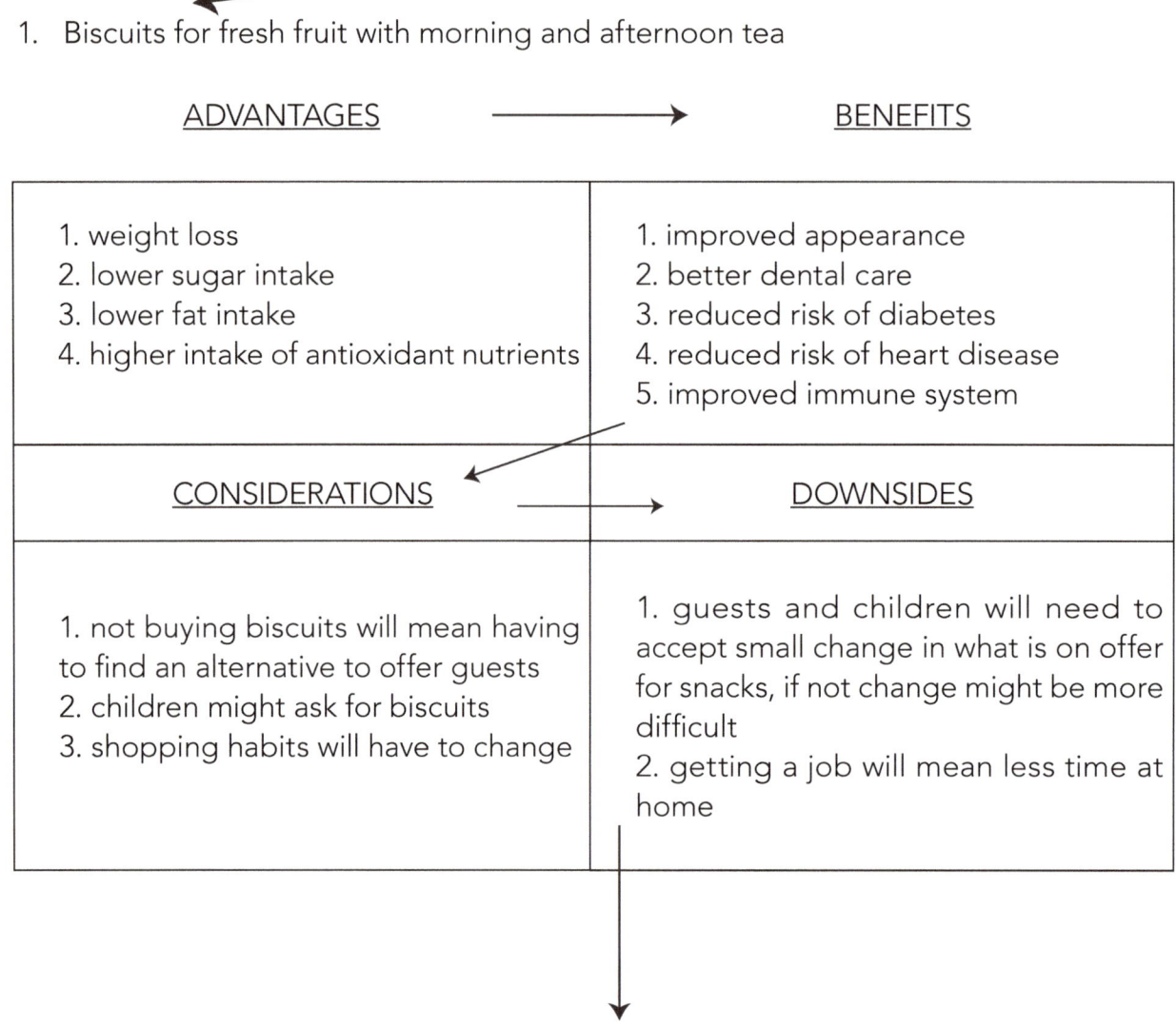

CHANGES

1.   Biscuits for fresh fruit with morning and afternoon tea

ADVANTAGES ⟶ BENEFITS

1. weight loss 2. lower sugar intake 3. lower fat intake 4. higher intake of antioxidant nutrients	1. improved appearance 2. better dental care 3. reduced risk of diabetes 4. reduced risk of heart disease 5. improved immune system
CONSIDERATIONS	DOWNSIDES
1. not buying biscuits will mean having to find an alternative to offer guests 2. children might ask for biscuits 3. shopping habits will have to change	1. guests and children will need to accept small change in what is on offer for snacks, if not change might be more difficult 2. getting a job will mean less time at home

CAN BE MITIGATED BY

1.   Educating children about nutrition
2.   Paying for a cleaner with money earned from a new job

In your learning groups, try a script of your own, this can begin with a script that a group member often uses themselves, one that several people have in common or one that you make up just for practice. Your facilitator will then hand you a fresh A-D chart, and you can practice transposing the positive story on to this. Later, you can try this with small changes in each of your own lives

You may now wish to take a few minutes to discuss this.

Group Discussion

WHOSE WORLD IS IT ANYWAY?

A well-known cleric, psychologist and advocator for the power of the creative mind, The late Dr Reg Barrett once said in a talk, given in Johannesburg, South Africa that "no one person, individually has ever changed the world. What some people have done, however, is change the attitude of the people in it. By changing your attitude towards the world, you change the world you live in, for you, forever".

We have now reached the end of this programme and the beginning of the rest of our lives. We have, together, found out how to make the best of ourselves, our health in the present and our health in the future. We now know how to make decisions effectively, and we know more about who we are and what we are capable of than we did when we began this programme. Now, without any prompt questions, the floor is open to you, the participants. Who is in charge of your life, and what are you going to do with it?

References

1. Crick F. The Astonishing Hypothesis. London: Simon and Schuster; 1994.
2. Levin J. God, Faith and Health. New York: John Wiley and Sons; 2001.
3. Islam MK, Merlo J, Kawachi I, Lindstrom M, Gerdtham UG. Social capital and health: Does egalitarianism matter? A literature review. International Journal for Equity in Health. Volume 5, 2006.
4. Olphen Jv, Schulz A, Israel B, et al. Religious Involvement, Social Support and Health Among African-American Women on the East Side of Detroit. Journal of General Internal Medicine. 2003;18:549-57.
5. DeHaven MJ, Hunter IB, Wilder L, Walton JW, Berry J. Health Programmes in Faith-Based Organisations: Are They Effective? American Journal of Public Health. 2004(94):1030-6.
6. Gautam R, Saito T, Kai I. Leisure and religious activity participation and mental health: gender analysis of older adults in Nepal. Biomed Central Public Health. Volume 7, 2007.
7. Szaflarski M, Ritchey PN, Leonard AC, et al. Modeling the Effects of Spirituality / Religion on Patients' Perceptions of Living with HIV/AIDS. Journal of General Internal Medicine. 2006;21:S28-38.
8. Daaleman TP, Perera S, Studenski SA. Religion, Spirituality and Health Status in Geriatric Outpatients. Annals of Family Medicine. Volume 2, 2004:49-53.
9. Ai AL, Peterson C, Bolling SF, Rodgers W. Depression, faith-based coping, and short-term postoperative global functioning in adult and older patients undergoing cardiac surgery. Journal of Psychosomatic Research. 2006(60):21-8.
10. Byrd RC. Positive therapeutic effects of intercessory prayer in a coronary care unit population. Southern Medical Journal. 1988;8:826-9.
11. Cohen N, Kehrl H, Berglund B, et al. Psychoneuroimmunology. Environmental Health Perspectives. 1997;105(2):527-9.
12. Davis MC, Zautra AJ, Smith B. Chronic Pain, Stress and the Dynamics of Affective Differentiation. Journal of Personality. Volume 72, 2004:1133-59.
13. Gralinski-Bakker JH, Hauser ST, Stott C, Billings RL, Allen JP. Markers of Resilience and Risk: Adult Lives in a Vulnerable Population. Research in Human Development. 2004;1(4):291-326.
14. Seligman M. Authentic Happiness. London: Nicholas Brealey Publishing; 2002.
15. Pert CB. Molecules of Emotion: Why You Feel the Way You Feel. New York: Scribner; 1998.
16. Byrne R. The Secret. New York: Beyond Words Publishing: Atria Books; 2006.
17. Watanabe E, Fukuda S, Shirakawa T. Effects among healthy subjects of the duration of regularly practising a guided imagery programme. Biomed Central Complementary and Alternative Medicine. Volume 5, 2005.
18. Hamilton C, Hinks S, Petticrew M. Arts for health: still searching for the Holy Grail. Journal of Epidemiology and Community Health. 2003;57:401-2.
19. Rogers MAM, Zaragoza-Lao E. Happiness and Children's Health: An Investigation of Art, Entertainment and Recreation. American Journal of Public Health. 2003;93(2):288-9.

20. Trent B. Art in the hospital: Treating the mind as well as the body. Canadian Medical Association Journal. 1986;135:1198-204.

21. Riley S. Art therapy with adolescents. Western Journal of Medicine. 2001;175:54-7.

22. Lowe G. Health-related effects of creative and expressive writing. Health Education. 2006;106(1):60-70.

23. Roux GMl. "Whistle While You Work": A Historical Account of Some Associations Among Music, Work and Health. American Journal of Public Health. Volume 95, 2005:1106-8.

24. Hilliard RE. Music Therapy in Hospice and Palliative Care: a Review of the Empirical Data. Complementary and Alternative Medicine. Volume 2, 2005:173-8.

25. Erkkila J, Gold C, Fachner J, Ala-Ruona E, Punkanen M, Vanhala M. The effect of improvisational music therapy on the treatment of depression: protocol for a randomised controlled trial. Biomed Central Psychiatry. Volume 8, 2008.

26. Romanelli F, Cain J, Smith KM. Emotional Intelligence as a Predictor of Academic and / or Professional Success. American Journal of Pharmaceutical Education. Volume 70, 2006.

Lightning Source UK Ltd.
Milton Keynes UK
UKHW050657021219
354499UK00011B/78/P

9 781984 592569